PRAISE FOR *RESHAPE YOUR LIFE*

"A very special book by a very special person. Written with wisdom, truth, and compassion, this book will inspire you to create your finest life."

—ROBIN SHARMA, #1 WORLDWIDE BESTSELLING AUTHOR OF *THE 5AM CLUB* AND *THE MONK WHO SOLD HIS FERRARI*

"Sometimes we are so desperate for change that we don't see the obvious signs pointing us to true happiness. *Reshape Your Life* will remind you that everything happens for a reason, and the pain you feel today is pointing you toward tomorrow's blessing. Thank you, Ali, for being so vulnerable about your journey and encouraging others to jump through fear into joy and daily gratitude."

—ROMA DOWNEY, ACTRESS, PRODUCER, AND BESTSELLING AUTHOR

"When I met Ali, she was just starting her journey to upgrade her health. She's been a master student and reshaped everything from her coffee habit to her daily intake of quality fats. She went all in with my Upgrade Labs facility in LA, where she used our tech to completely rewire her health at a cellular level. Ali, you didn't settle and you are worth it, and your book will greatly help so many people to upgrade their lives too."

—DAVE ASPREY, FATHER OF BIOHACKING, FOUNDER OF BULLETPROOF, AND *NEW YORK TIMES* BESTSELLING AUTHOR

"Ali Landry is the real deal. The most authentic, genuine women I know. She is driven when it comes to her health and wellness and family. I am so proud to call her my friend."

—GARCELLE BEAUVAIS, ACTRESS AND TELEVISION PERSONALITY

"Ali Landry is, quite simply, the magic in the room. Sure, she lights it up—that's a given. The remarkable magic about Ali is that she somehow figures out how to shine her light directly on you so that you can finally see—and celebrate—what you have had inside you all along! I always (half) joke with my husband that I dream about a day I can just follow Ali around and do whatever she says. Thanks to this extraordinary book, I have that day and then some! With Ali, dreams really do come true."

—GAIL BECKER, FOUNDER OF CAULIPOWER

RESHAPE
YOUR LIFE

RESHAPE YOUR LIFE

DON'T SETTLE BECAUSE YOU ARE WORTH IT

ALI LANDRY

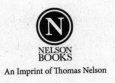

NELSON
BOOKS

An Imprint of Thomas Nelson

ISBN 978-1-4002-3511-7 (eBook)
ISBN 978-1-4002-3510-0 (HC)

Library of Congress Control Number: 2022948478

Printed in the United States of America
23 24 25 26 27 LBC 5 4 3 2 1

This book is dedicated to every woman who believes she is worthy of a life that is fulfilling and spectacular. My prayer, from my heart to yours, is that this book meets you exactly where you are.

CONTENTS

CONTENTS

THE PERFECT TIME FOR A RESHAPE

*We cannot become what we want
by remaining what we are.*

MAX DEPREE

Reshape:

(verb) to give a new form or orientation to

(noun) a life-altering event that changes the
course of your life or transforms you

Hi! I am Ali Landry, wife, mom, daughter, sister, actress, host, entrepreneur, and wellness explorer—like so many of us, I wear many hats. Tapping into my own greatness, recognizing my superpower, and encouraging other women to do it for themselves, drives my dedication to see all women reshape the areas of life that are no longer serving them. I believe it is never too late to pivot or change to create a life you love. It's all about finding the best resources, education, tools, and community to take action and fight for it, never settling for less than you deserve.

I love seeing a woman completely thrive. When I see a woman not living with desire, joy, or fulfillment, it breaks my heart. So often, we as women get stuck—we get stuck in relationships that diminish us, jobs that don't suit us, eating habits that deplete us, schedules that exhaust us, mindsets that steal our vision, and routines that no longer serve us. It's not like any of us get stuck on purpose. Life happens. But as poet Maya Angelou famously said to Oprah Winfrey, "When you know better, you do better."[1]

I have chosen to educate myself and assess every area of my life over the last twenty years in an attempt to build the very best version of myself every day. What about you? Are you going to face what needs to change and choose to custom design a life that you love? When you recognize an area of your life that needs a reshape, either big or small, what is your self-talk? I hope you tell yourself that you are worth it.

God created each of us on purpose. I hope my reshape experience will inspire you for yours.

What Is a Reshape?

We've all had those times when we realize a certain area of life is no longer serving us. We must make a decision to either settle or step up and figure it out. These are seasons of reshaping, and while some are more significant than others, all are important to our quality of life—and to who we ultimately become.

In this book I'll share some of my own reshapes. These include defining moments in my life, some very public and some intensely private, all of them pivotal. While some were life changing and beautiful, others were extremely uncomfortable, even heartbreaking. They challenged me and pushed me to step into life at a whole new level. Because of them, I was forced to do a deep dive into myself and learn to approach life differently. These moments were transformational for me because I did the work, reshaping what wasn't working for me anymore. Honestly, the vision for this book came from these reshape moments.

Rude Awakening

What started me on this journey was landing my dream job, a daily syndicated talk show called *Hollywood Today Live*. I'd dreamed of hosting a talk show for years, and this seemed a perfect fit for me. On paper the schedule looked great for a busy wife and mom of three. I'd start early in the morning, get in a workout, then be available for my family in the afternoons. The reality was quite different from what I'd imagined. While it seemed like I should have been on top of the world, thrilled, living my best life, in reality I was exhausted! I was losing my hair, I had poor digestion, low sex drive, mild depression . . . the list goes on. I felt so off. I didn't feel sick enough to see a doctor, but at the same time I knew that something wasn't right. My girlfriends passed it off as aging, but that didn't sit well with me. I wasn't going to settle. So I dug down deep. I found the fire inside of me to get to the bottom of how I was feeling. Then I got to work! The results were nothing short of transformational. I'll share the full story later, in chapter 3, but for now just know that I found the vibrancy in life I so desired. That's what I believe every woman deserves. And I am determined to help you get to yours too.

The desire to reach the full potential of who I was created to be is foundational for how I have built my life, both personally and professionally. When trials come, as they inevitably do, I walk into the situation knowing I'm not going to stay stuck and let circumstances dictate my future. I have a mindset of striving to never settle.

Reshaping is not a one-time thing. It is a journey. Whether your heart, mind, soul, or health need a change, you are worth the effort to spend the time and find the resources you need to create a life you love and fully live into your purpose. I have worked to build a community of people who feel like sunshine and who recognize my superpowers. I would love to be part of your community, to cheer you on, help you with your own reshape, and support your dreams and visions for your life.

My encouragement to you is this: do not settle, because you are worth it. We only get one life, and we should make it a masterpiece.

The Birth of RE/SHAPE

I created my lifestyle company RE/SHAPE to build a community where women could find the education, resources, tools, wellness experts, game-changing products, and inspiration for a total reshape—heart, mind, soul, and health.

When I started down the road to reshape my health, it was a big task to research and find the information I was looking for that could help me take responsibility for figuring out and fixing what was going on. At the time, I would've loved to have found one place with a trusted, curated, broad scope of resources that could guide me to achieve my goals and reach my reshape a little faster and more efficiently. That's why I went to work and built the lifestyle company RE/SHAPE.

I love to research and become knowledgeable about products and services. Many of my girlfriends don't have the time, don't know where to look, and don't know the questions to ask. I enjoy being in the hot seat, asking the questions, trying the treatments, and being the guinea pig so I can report back. I will give most anything one try, and taking you on the adventure with me makes it all the more fun and worthwhile.

I have worked through some major health issues and dealt with tragedy, loss, heartbreak, and betrayal, all of which catapulted me into a necessary reshape to move my life beyond my circumstances. I was determined not to let difficulties define me. I have experienced tremendous growth personally, along with an increased internal strength after doing the necessary work. As women, we are at our best when we are supporting one another. My hope is that this book will meet you where you are and be a guiding light for your own personal reshape exploration.

Do You Need a Reshape?

So, what about you? What areas of your life need a reshape?

I look at overall wellness and thriving in life from an integrative perspective. Our hearts, minds, souls, and health are intertwined.

It's like my friend and mentor Robin Sharma says: the mindset, heartset, healthset, and soulset are all connected. As we grow in heart, mind, health, and soul, that releases pressure in all the other areas of our life. As you step back and look at any area you'd like to reshape, recognize the need to evaluate and touch on each of these most intimate areas. Often addressing one area of struggle will trigger struggle in the other areas. We can't reshape one area without looking at another. I'm not saying to reshape everything at once; just be aware and notice how one area impacts others.

The patterns we create for ourselves can often become the primary factor when we get off track and part of our life begins to drag us down. We get into patterns for all sorts of reasons and, as we know, patterns are hard to break. To counteract patterns, I am a big fan of routines—specific routines to help stay on track, make the most of the day, and bring purpose to life. Patterns and routines are different in my eyes—while patterns can happen by accident, routines are intentional.

What is your daily pattern of life? How are the weekdays and weekends treating you? Are you waking up exhausted? Does life hit you on a Monday morning like a Mack truck? Or do you have a morning routine in place that serves your overall wellness so you feel energized and ready to take on the world? My routine was waking up, hitting the snooze button, having my kids run into the room, and hustling to make breakfast and get them to school, followed by full days of work and then family responsibilities. That brought me to end my day with just getting through dinner, getting kids to bed, and watching Netflix on my iPad in bed with baked Cheetos until I dozed off. Spending months in this pattern is only going to bring us to one place: completely agitated and unsettled. It was a pattern I didn't set out to have; nonetheless, this pattern became my daily life, and it came from the circumstances I was facing at the time. I decided it was impacting not only me but my family and the atmosphere in our home. I'd had enough. I made a commitment to myself to figure out a better sleep strategy and a morning routine. When I put these two systems in place, my life completely transitioned to become more manageable in every area, and I no longer felt drained or unmotivated before the day began.

How is your health? I can tell you, mine needed a major overhaul. I was struggling in some areas and was just living with it, thinking problems would go away or I would get to them at some later point. It was only when I started working on the daily talk show *Hollywood Today Live* that all of my issues became significantly elevated. It forced me to look for the support I needed (I'll dive into this more in the next chapter). Why do we as women always put ourselves in last place on our list of priorities? I think it is our nature to serve others, but not taking care of ourselves impacts not only us but everyone around us. How many times have we been told this?

Have you, like me, spent too much time at different moments in life focused on that magic number? Have you thought that if you could just lose X number of pounds you would be happy? I have, and it's a really uncomfortable truth for me to admit. It makes me sad when I realize that I let that thought creep in. The funny thing is, I have hit the magic number that I dreamt about before. I honestly thought that all of a sudden when I saw that number on the scale, everything in my life would be unicorns and rainbows. But it wasn't. I was still at times sad, unsatisfied with life, and full of anxiety. I should have known better; life doesn't mysteriously transform when a certain number shows up on a scale. Choosing to love your whole self at every turn on your journey is a choice—a choice only you can make. Sometimes this choice requires a deliberate reshape across all areas of your life: heart, mind, soul, and health.

How is your environment? Does it give you life or drain your life?

I am big on clearing out the clutter around our home because it not only makes me feel restless to look at it and know I need to do something about it, but it makes my mind even more cluttered, leaving less space for thinking, planning, dreaming, and anything creative I want to do. This is an area most of us would benefit from reshaping and implementing a routine that helps us clean up the clutter around our environment regularly—every week, every month, or once per quarter. You can't wait for spring-cleaning time to deal with your house, your car, and your mind.

How is your overall look? How are you presenting yourself to the world? Have you lost your mojo a little or maybe lost it altogether? Our outside appearance is often an indicator of what is going on in the inside. Are you overwhelmed with life? Do you just not care? Is your wardrobe not fitting like it used to? Are you in survival mode and it's all you can do to pull it together for yourself or your family? I think many of us have been there. I want to encourage you to find a sliver of time each week to take care of you. We all need time to get ourselves together so we can look and feel good. If you make the time for a mini reshape in this area, the benefit will come back tenfold across every area of your life.

How is your time management? Are you feeling exhausted every day? If so, from what? Are you spending too much time on social media, watching the news, or streaming your favorite show while disconnected from the people around you? How is any of this enhancing your life and your future? Often when we get exhausted we fall into these cycles of living, surviving, and just going through the motions. Because I've been there, I now do my best to stay very aware of myself, and if I am going down that path, I try to be quick to nip it. The longer we keep to these patterns, the harder they are to reshape.

Maybe your career choice is running you into a dead end and you've lost interest. Perhaps you are in an unhealthy relationship for whatever reason. Do you need to step up your fitness game? Have you made the time for your passion projects? Do you need to update your skincare and makeup, since, as we age, we need to switch up our products? Or do you just simply need to change up your snacks and sweeteners to find a healthier option like I needed to?

It can be hard, emotional, even terrifying to face the need for change, but you are worth it. Look in the mirror and be honest with yourself about what is working in your life—and what is not. What needs to change? What *is* working for you is a big indicator. You know what makes you happy and feeling your best. It's time to write down your reshape goals, find your tools, put accountability in place, and get going. I'll help you along the way. Think of where your life could be one week from now or one month from now, even one year from now. All it takes is one small change at a time.

Natural-Born Sharer

I think each of us has been created with certain natural gifts. It's very important to recognize those gifts so we can honor ourselves and who God made us to be. For example, one of my gifts is connecting with people. I have made a career out of it. I firmly believe that when you speak from the heart, you touch the heart. It's about being authentic, honest, and meeting each other where we are.

Connecting with people, especially women, gives me energy—it always has. I love to learn people's stories; it actually helps me reflect on my own life. One of my favorite opportunities through RE/SHAPE is sharing with other women about the resources I have found that have been total game changers in my life. There is so much clutter out there in the media that I get so excited when I find those gems. I want to tell the whole world. I have found over the years that women in my circle of friends and business colleagues often come to me and ask for advice on relationships; they want to know what green juice I'm drinking, my skincare routine, my latest health hack, and even how I style my wardrobe. I love to share with them about all these things, from the deep emotions of the heart to my favorite lip gloss. When we are trying our best to live a full and meaningful life, all these things are important.

I'm an open book, literally—it's all here in these pages! I'm sharing with you some of the essential tools, resources, and wellness strategies I have gathered along the way. It's been an incredible experience for me to meet, talk with, and be coached by leading experts in the wellness space. I am bringing you all the guidance, protocols, products, and practices they provided to me in hopes that it will serve you in a powerful way, like it did for me.

While none of us has traveled the exact same road in life, so many of our experiences and feelings are similar. Sometimes our reshapes can be fast, like how putting blackout electrical tape on electronic lights in your bedroom can quickly upgrade your sleep experience. Other reshapes are so deep that we need to prepare every part of ourselves to go there and release whatever has our soul stuck. Reshaping is an ongoing process over the course of our lives. Genuinely knowing yourself, creating a certain mindset, living with intention, and being present in your life is fundamental. We are going to cover it all here.

Face the Fear

A few years back I met Tony Robbins with my husband when we attended his conference for my husband's business. I remember when Tony said to an audience of thousands that "everything you want is on the other side of fear." Isn't that so true? Some of the best experiences and memories in my life have come from just going for it, whether I felt ready or not—even pushing through any anxious feelings I've had from time to time. Tony's statement seems simple enough, but in reality, fear keeps many of us from living—I mean really living—life in full color. In different ways and for different reasons, fear has been one area in my life that I've had to conquer. This is where my daily practice of prayer and meditation comes in. I can release any fear in my heart and in my mind. After all, fear is not real. Your feelings, emotions, and history are real, but they are all areas where you can make a shift and reshape. Fear can be debilitating, but *we* are not about to let that happen here!

There is so much to explore together. If you are ready to reshape one small area of your life or fully transform and create a life you love, this book is for you. As I share some of my story with you, we are going to jump right into the matters of the heart, mind, soul, and health. We are going to get in there to do some big-time self-evaluation. I hope you will use this book as a guide. So get your highlighter and get ready.

We'll start with a story that begins in a small town, where everyone knows each other by name.

CHAPTER 1

SMALL-TOWN GIRL AND A CAREER RESHAPE

*Be who God meant you to be and
you will set the world on fire.*

SAINT CATHERINE OF SIENA

Los Angeles, California, has been my home for years. I got my break in the entertainment business here. It's where I fell in love with my husband. It's where I gave birth to our three beautiful children. We've made lots of wonderful memories in LA with dear friends. There's no denying the beauty of this place; after all, it is one of the most famous cities in the world. For me, there's nothing like sinking your toes in the sand while the waves of the Pacific crash and foam at your feet, then driving just a short way to the mountains for a sunset dinner. LA is also recognized by most of the world as the entertainment capital, home to Hollywood and all the glitz and glamour that comes with it.

But I'm from a very different LA—LA for Louisiana. These days in California, I'm never far from Interstate 10. If I were to hop on that freeway and drive east for a few days, I'd wind up at the Henderson, Louisiana, exit, only three minutes from the house I grew up in.

My Louisiana Home

"Just a small-town girl . . ." That iconic first line of that classic Journey song instantly transports me to 1997, the year I moved to LA. I'd slide their CD into my CD player and sing along (off key) at the top of my lungs on my way to casting calls and auditions. Traffic in LA was tricky even then, so I'd carefully map out my routes using the *Thomas Guide*. We didn't have Waze or iPhones or even GPS yet, so planning was crucial if I wanted to arrive early. All the while I'd be humming Journey's song under my breath.

I still love that song. Steve Perry might as well be singing about me; that's how I still think of myself: "just a small-town girl" if ever there was one. And the chorus perfectly captured what I learned growing up in Louisiana: don't stop believing.

Cajun Roots

I grew up on the border of Breaux Bridge and Cecilia, two very small towns in southwest Louisiana. If I could take you there now, you'd see how the land stretches out forever into the horizon, the distances defined by varying shades of green hinting at crops—soybean, corn, and sugarcane—fed by the muddy waters of the Bayou Teche. I'd point out the crumbling silos from the old sugarcane mill. We used to lay under those ancient oak trees—majestic, mysterious, with their strong roots twisting, turning into the soil, their branches dripping with Spanish moss. Stepping under their canopy is like stepping into a different world.

The air is thick and smells of fresh-cut grass. It tends to rain every day, though sometimes just a drizzle. There's nothing like walking to the end of a dock as a light rain falls on the bayou, the fish and tadpoles breaking the surface of the water to say hello. Church bells ring out the hours. A symphony of birds and insects plays all day, rising as night falls.

The pace of life is a little slower there. Everybody knows everybody. We Cajuns are known for our hospitality, so when you run into someone you know, you stop and visit, unlike in Los Angeles where everyone is in such a hurry. We'd visit my family. There'd be no need to call ahead—doors in my town were always open and there was likely a meal to feed ten simmering on the stove.

That's the way I grew up, close to all my family. Some of my sweetest memories are of running from yard to yard, playing hide and seek. You see, both sets of my grandparents lived on two large pieces of land that they separated between their children. We lived on my dad's family's land, so I spent a lot of time with Mom Landry, my dad's mom. I loved the stories she would tell me about days gone by, her weathered hands telling a story of their own. I loved hearing about what came before me, stories of humble beginnings and hardworking people connected to the land, their faith, and their community, always showing up to help each other out.

My dad is one of twelve children. My mom is one of eight. All our family lived close by, so I grew up with lots of cousins—forty-five first cousins in all—plus my brother and sister. Every Friday my grandmother would cook for the whole family. My aunts would go to my mom's beauty salon to get their hair done. And then they'd walk next door to my grandmother's house to have lunch and spend the day together. Fridays during the summer were my favorite days. My cousins and I played while all the women were in the kitchen helping prepare lunch—shrimp stews, crawfish étouffée, fish coubion, rice and gravy, or gumbo. We'd gather in the afternoon and share that delicious meal. It was heaven.

My family's land stretched across several acres. My parents' house was right next door to my grandmother's house. We had the run of the place. It was a magical childhood. Nature was my playground. A classic tomboy, I was always running around outside, climbing trees, and leading my cousins on wild adventures. During harvest season, we'd dive into grain bins filled with soybeans, pretending to swim in the ocean. I rode my bike, jumped on the trampoline, played in the barn, and dug in the dirt for treasures.

Running around barefoot, climbing mossy oak trees, traipsing around in the creeks and bayous, watching chickens hatch from eggs, watching the rise and fall of the bayou—that was how I spent much of my childhood. It's funny because in the wellness world I am in now, this is called "forest bathing" or "grounding." For us it was just growing up in the country.

I could tell when rain was coming by the scent of the air. From a young age, I saw how living things are always changing, growing, moving. Nothing alive stays the same. That was something I knew in my bones. It was a thrilling thought, especially for someone like me with a big imagination.

Landry Life

My dad worked in the oil fields—seven days on, seven days off. So I was used to not having him there all the time. When he was home, we totally catered to him. I never heard my parents argue or raise their voices to each other. Never. He was and still is a bit of a homebody—hardworking and all about family. Sugar cane ripened in the field behind our house. I can remember my dad and I walking out to the field on a hot day. He'd pull out the knife he always had in his pocket and cut a piece of that perfectly sweet ripe sugarcane. I can still taste it. Dad was most comfortable out there on the land or at home. He was famously good-looking and known to be a brawler back in his younger days, but he's still one of the gentlest and kindest men I've ever met.

My mom is the social one. Everyone knew if you wanted something done, you called Renella. She could and still can do anything she sets her mind to. I think this was my first lesson in mind reshaping. My mom was an entrepreneur and ran a thriving business as a hairdresser in her little salon built on the side of our house. It gave her a perfect work-life balance. If you've seen *Steel Magnolias*, that was basically my mom's beauty shop. Nothing fancy—just three chairs, two hair washing basins, and a couple of dryers. She could go back and forth from the salon to our house to check on whatever she had cooking, usually rice and gravy, and then tell us to pick up our rooms. She could go back and forth and never miss one beat. She worked all day, so she was always busy, but she was always, always there to check on us. She would run into the house quickly, grab a bite, and then go back into the shop to take care of her customers. And we kids were always in and out. I can still hear that screen door opening and closing, opening and closing. She was such a wonderful example of a strong, confident woman who took care of everyone she loved. All that I am is because of my mother. She is a creative genius who runs circles around me, energy-wise, even to this day, which is why I knew when I was in my midforties and exhausted that something was off. She shows up in the world in the most selfless ways for her friends and family and will always be my superwoman.

The Mindset that I Could Do Anything

From a young age I was always competitive. Maybe that comes from being the firstborn and wanting to excel at everything. I wanted to do it all. From the time I could walk, I took dance classes and did gymnastics. It seemed like every little girl where I grew up went to dance class. I went to Miss Linda first, and then Miss Liz. Then, as I got older, I signed up for every sport that was offered in my area. I played softball, volleyball, I was on a competitive cheerleading squad, I was head cheerleader at school, part of student council—I loved it all. I'm not saying I was great at all these things, but I definitely wanted to give them a good go. I loved the adventure of trying something new. Competing gave me the opportunity to see and imagine living outside my little town. It was my window to the wider world.

Soon I was competing in pageants. There are lots of opportunities because Louisiana is famous for festivals and parades, the most famous being Mardi Gras in New Orleans. But there are so many more that celebrate everything from music to history to food. Our state is separated into church parishes instead of counties. Many towns have a specific crop they're known for, and there's a special festival for every area's special crop. Everyone participates. The town's streets are closed off and there's lots of live music, plenty of booths selling local fare, and a big parade. Breaux Bridge is known for crawfish, so our local festival is the Crawfish Festival, but there are all kinds of festivals throughout the state: the Frog Festival in Rayne, the Rice Festival in Crowley, the Sugarcane Festival in New Iberia, and hundreds more. Honestly, we Louisianians take full advantage of any excuse to have a party and gather as a community. And how can you have a festival and a parade without a queen? There's always a "Little Miss Pincher," a "Miss Étouffée," a "Crawfish Queen" (that was my sister). It's part of the culture and a way to celebrate your heritage.

Though pageants were a part of my childhood, they weren't my dream. My dream was travel, to explore the world and other cultures and to make a name for myself doing something I loved. I wasn't sure what that meant, but I knew it would take me out of my beloved Louisiana. So, after high school graduation, I enrolled at USL—now known as the University of Louisiana at Lafayette—to study journalism and marketing and take on the world. My professors quickly burst my bubble. They told us our first jobs out of college would most likely be interning or being an assistant to on-camera talent until we "learned the ropes." I didn't see myself doing that. I thought, *I need to figure out a way to skip a few rungs on this job ladder.* After all, I had a big vision and was determined to make it happen.

I'd competed in enough pageants to know that Miss Louisiana USA got to travel around the state and meet all kinds of sponsors and new people. I figured if I competed and won, I'd be able to make enough connections to travel up the corporate ladder a little quicker. No delivering coffee for this small-town girl! I was determined not to let someone else's idea of a career path become my future. I knew there was another way, and I was laser focused on getting there.

I talked to my mom about it. She immediately said, "Ali, do you really want to do this? We are so busy right now!" She knew the pageant system required a lot of work because we'd done them together before. But I was determined. I told her I'd do all the work. She gave in and supported me. When I won Miss Louisiana, I was wearing a beautiful black velvet gown that my mom and I designed, made by Mrs. Janice Duplichien Thibodeaux.

As Miss Louisiana USA, I traveled around the state. And, sure enough, during that time, a seismic data company based in Houston, Texas, offered me a job in public relations. I thought, *This is great!* I felt satisfied because that was the goal. I'd accomplished what I'd set out to do.

The Stakes Rise

As Miss Louisiana USA, it was part of my obligation to represent Louisiana in the Miss USA Pageant. I saw that for the opportunity it was. Maybe I could do something with this beyond securing a good job—I might be able to help other women as well.

I had already accomplished my initial goal, but as in anything I do, I was going to do it with my whole self. So, I arrived for the two weeks of pageant competition with a positive mindset. I said, "If I am here, I am here to win." Then I had a reality check. The other women had brought hair pieces and huge wardrobes completely planned out for every day. These girls were not playing games, and I wondered if I had prepared enough. Self-doubt started to creep in. I quickly realized I needed to flip the switch on the way I was thinking. I knew that if I wanted to stay in the game, I could not let these thoughts of feeling less-than affect me. In other words, I was aware that these thoughts were passing through my mind, but I was not going to identify with them personally.

The rigorous pageant schedule included rehearsals all day every day, leading up to the live event. And every evening we'd go to cocktail events or dinners, greeting sponsors, area business leaders, and supporters. I loved meeting interesting, engaging people, but it was an intense schedule for all of us.

As the days went by, I could see some of the girls starting to compare themselves with each other—a rabbit hole that I'd almost fallen down a few days prior. I could see a bit of jealousy forming, and the pressures of the competition really began to wear on their spirits. I thought, *This is not good. They are going to start falling off because they can't stay in the mental game of the competition.* I knew I didn't have the best dress or the best body, I probably wasn't as well prepared as most, and I wasn't that used to public speaking, but I also knew that I was uniquely me. I was going to put blinders on, stay in my lane, and "do me." I chose to focus on the positive, knowing that I had as good a chance as anyone else and I was going to give it my all. So, yeah—why not me?!

> Don't be concerned with how others define you. When they define you, they are limiting themselves, so it's their problem.
>
> *Eckhart Tolle*

With the mounting pressures as we came closer to the final night of the competition, I somehow managed to stay focused. It was a huge mental challenge and exercise. Then, the night before the competition, I felt myself getting tired, not only physically but mentally. I was doubting myself again, and I needed to quickly come up with a plan to get back on track. So I decided to play hooky from the events of the evening. I stayed behind in the room when my roommate left. I drew a bath, lay in the tub, closed my eyes, and practiced visualization. Visualization, simply put, helps to prepare you to respond to a situation before it happens. It also helps to achieve your goals by conditioning your brain to see, hear, and feel the success in your mind. That night in the tub I visualized being on the stage. I visualized every aspect of that final night. How I felt on the stage with the lights and the hum of the crowd. I visualized God's light shining through me. I visualized being happy and calm and representing all those in southwest Louisiana who were cheering me on. I visualized the crown being put on my head, but there was something else that was blocking me, standing in my way, creating fear in my mind. You see, during rehearsals we learned that the final three contestants would be in a clear glass booth. They'd wear headphones so they couldn't hear the first girl who went out to answer a live question from a judge. The other two would watch from the booth, unable to hear, but they would be able to see everything. I was sure I'd been calm and cool up until then. I thought, *If I'm in the top three, having to watch from that glass soundproof booth, I don't know if I can make it. I think my nerves would completely take over!* So I prayed, "God, if you want this for me, and I am in the top three, let me be called first."

The next night, when they announced the top three, I was called first. An incredible peace washed over me. My exact prayer had been answered. I'd prayed in such specific detail. Now it was like God winked at me, assuring me that we were in this together. I whispered, "Thank you, God!" As I answered the final question, I didn't feel rattled at all.

The producers orchestrate the entire evening to this crescendo, a supercharged moment. Everything from the music to the lighting to the staging to the commercial breaks—all of it is a buildup of tension to that question, "Who will be crowned Miss USA?"

I was standing with Miss Kansas when the announcer said, "Ali Landry, Miss Louisiana, you are the new Miss USA!"

Winning Miss USA changed the course of my life.

Community Over Crown

What had started as a desire to skip a couple of steps on the job ladder turned out to be such a proud moment for my town and my community. This was so much bigger than me. In that moment when I was being crowned Miss USA and given a bouquet of roses, in all that excitement, all I could think about was my family and friends gathered back home in each other's houses, watching on TV, and how happy they'd be. I knew they'd be jumping up and down and hugging each other, and it was true! Most of my extended family had gathered in one home, which is not rare for Cajuns because they will come together for anything, and the local TV station was there, broadcasting live. When it was announced that I won, they were ecstatic. The whole town was.

All of Louisiana was so supportive of me. Everyone was so proud. Honestly, to this day that gives me more joy than winning ever did.

I was then swept up into the world of being Miss USA. The morning after I won I had breakfast with my parents, and then, with only the clothes I had for the two weeks of competition, I immediately flew to Los Angeles, deboarded, was ushered into a towncar, and taken directly to the set of the *George and Alana* talk show where I was literally in my little interview suit from the competition. This was a whole new world for me. I buckled up and got ready for the ride.

After a few months of getting used to my new job title, I had the amazing opportunity to go back home to Louisiana for a home-coming event. I can't tell you how excited I was to go home and see everyone. It was only to be a two-day trip, but I would take it. I just needed to get back and ground myself in my Louisiana roots, see all the people who'd loved and supported me personally, and thank them from the bottom of my heart. It felt like a nearly impossible task, but I was determined to do it.

Fortunately, a Breaux Bridge Chamber board member and family friend, Ray Pellerin, and Kris Dugas, director of Breaux Bridges chamber of commerce, stepped in to plan my homecoming with thirty or so community leaders and coordinators from each venue and over two hundred Breaux Bridge and Cecilia volunteers. I'm still amazed at what they accomplished on short notice and I am forever grateful. For me that time was about honoring the people who'd poured so much into my life. It was about family, faith, and community.

Since flying commercially into New Orleans would cost precious time, my incredible hometown team arranged a locally owned private jet to fly me straight into Lafayette's tiny airport. The biggest surprise of all was that my mom and godfather, Anthony "Tanny" Hebert, were on that plane to pick me up. My godfather was one of the most influential male figures in my life besides my own father. He just had a way with people. When you were with him, he made you feel like you were the most important person in the room. Everyone who knew him loved him, and he had been diagnosed with cancer earlier that year. That trip was the last time I saw his beautiful smile and felt the love in his giant hugs. As we exited the plane, we were greeted by a huge crowd. It felt like every able-bodied person from the area was invited! Stepping off that plane was surreal. I saw so many smiling, proud faces. That beautiful welcome made me realize that the most precious gift you give someone is your time and for them to feel seen and loved.

After I greeted as many people as I could in the airplane hangar, Kris told me it was time to go. I thanked everyone, said goodbye, then got on a coach to travel to the next event. On the way, we saw hand-painted signs and banners all over town that said, "Welcome Home, Ali! We love you!" My face was even on a billboard on I-10, the highway I had traveled many times as a younger woman, daydreaming about my future. That highway now connected my two LAs.

> See the light in others, and treat them as if that is all you see.
>
> *Dr. Wayne Dyer*

One of our first stops was the Acadian Village Chapel where we visited a Special Olympics group. Then we visited my elementary school, my high school, and my college—the University of Louisiana at Lafayette. I thanked my teachers and coaches, then spoke to the students and urged them to stay true to their values and who they are. The local kindergartners sang "God Bless America"—and there wasn't a dry eye in the place.

The homecoming parade was bigger than the Crawfish Festival! The loop around Breaux Bridge was packed with people. There was great Cajun music and great food for all to enjoy, but my focus was on connecting with the people. I handed out hundreds if not thousands of American flags and signed photos. At one point the parade stopped in front of the Breaux Bridge itself, where a photographer took a picture of me with the local Brownies, Girl Scouts, and school children. To this day when I go back home, I often see that photo hanging on the wall of local businesses and shops, and it still brings tears to my eyes in humility and gratitude.

Time stopped for me during that trip back home. I connected as best I could with each soul I came in contact with. My heart was full of gratitude, especially during my stop at the USS *Kidd* where I visited with veterans. My grandfather had served in the military, so I've always had a special place in my heart for our nation's men and women in uniform. I got a chance to express my thanks, and then, to my surprise, they gave me a twenty-one-gun salute. That was beyond anything I'd ever experienced. Our final stop was the governor's office for one final, historic meeting. The sheriff's department had blocked off all the exits on Interstate 10 so we could make it in time. The planning team had timed it so that I'd seen literally thousands of people in just two days. We covered a lot of miles in that coach!

When my narrow window of time in Louisiana was over, I got back on that private jet to head back to Las Vegas for the Miss Universe Pageant. I was not alone. My family, the homecoming planning committee, and several other friends came along. I wish I had a picture of all of them checking in to the hotel. I believe we Cajuns outnumbered the women in the Miss Universe pageant!

To this day, when I go home, people will come up to me and say, "Ali! You never forgot where you came from!" That's pretty much one of the greatest compliments I could get. I will always be that small-town girl in my heart. Louisiana will always be running through my veins.

Those intense days of homecoming changed something in me. I can remember praying the words of Martin Luther King Jr's famous quote, "Use me, God. Show me how to take who I am, who I want to be, and what I can do, and use it for a purpose greater than myself."[2]

It was humbling to realize that I was now in the public eye. I could see how much my being crowned Miss USA meant to so many people, and I felt a huge responsibility, but I was still not sure what that actually meant for me moving forward. All I knew for sure was that it was part of God's plan for my life, and I had to figure out how to honor him.

Destination: Hollywood

Miss Universe, the company, is based in Los Angeles, so, as Miss USA, I was required to live there during my reign. Thanks to my homecoming experience, I was more in touch than ever with my small-town roots, but I was ready to reshape my life in new ways. I knew LA was going to be the next chapter of my life. At first I was totally overwhelmed by the city and missed my home and family terribly. I knew this was where I needed to be, though. I would surrender to this opportunity. In LA, there was a whole new world of possibilities that I had never even considered for myself. It was scary but it was also exciting.

I just needed to channel my mom's can-do mindset. I would not stop believing.

Women Who Inspire

I'm proud of the woman I am today and the one I'm still becoming. I've experienced a lot, but I know that who I am is bound together with where I'm from. I do consider myself, at the end of the day, truly a small-town girl.

There are so many women who came before me in my life—women who set examples for me in how they showed up for one another. They were my greatest teachers—not always by their words, but more by their actions. They also taught me not to dim my own light to make others feel comfortable; when we as women shine, we lift each other up! When friends dream big and fearlessly, it's good not just for one but for all of us. Most of all they taught me what loyalty and love look like in action.

What I didn't know growing up is that Breaux Bridge, Louisiana, was founded by a woman. The very place I grew up—the place that built me—was built by a woman! Scholastique Picou Breaux was widowed at thirty-three, a mom to five children. Can you imagine? She had a vision for a town. She drew up plans that included a school, a church, and a diagram for all our streets. That town became Breaux Bridge. What a brave, strong, creative woman she must have been!

These days, when I go back, I visit her statue to pay homage. I get goosebumps thinking about it. Things didn't always go Scholastique Picou Breaux's way, but she did something amazing with what she'd been given as we all have that choice. She made her life a masterpiece. That's the kind of small-town girl I want to be.

At this point in my life, this is something I think about often. *What is my purpose?* Purpose is your why. This personal sense of purpose guides and fills up your heart. It gives you a sense of direction. Yes, it is a big question—but one worth asking, and answering. Your purpose is unique to you. It can be related to talents or your skill set or that thing that lights that fire inside of you. I believe it is connected to your joy. It's your reason for being—why you get up in the morning. It's more about the long game than short-term goals. And sometimes your purpose may change throughout your life. I believe tapping into mind shape, heart shape, and health shape can help you find your purpose. It's truly the reason I'm so passionate about helping you find your own reshape.

RESHAPE WRAP-UP

When you look at where you are now in your life, can you track much of it back to your childhood? Each of us experiences childhood differently, but nevertheless, childhood sets us on a course for the future. We can look back and identify good times and those that may have been more difficult—all of them the building blocks for a life. The beautiful part about this time in our lives is that we are in control of how we are going to let the experiences of our younger years shape our lives today.

The idea of having faith like a child can certainly get clouded as we move through life. The fundamental truth of that statement remains real. It's never too late to dream and create a vision for your life. You are worth the effort of going after anything you want and squeezing every experience out of your life that you can imagine for yourself.

Find the resolve within yourself to stay determined, be persistent, and recognize that you have everything it takes to accomplish any-thing you see for yourself—that is the ultimate goal for any of us. Do your best to not let discouragement get the better of you. The path to get where you want to go may not look like you thought it would, and the final destination may not be the actual vision you saw when you started on the journey, but I believe with all my heart that God allows you to arrive where he wants you. Even if you have to walk the entire road alone, be determined to maximize every ounce of potential you have: you are worth the time, the planning, and any tears it takes to get there.

RESHAPE MOVES

1. Identity your belief system and what was birthed in you from your history. Embrace who you are and where you come from—it is part of the fabric of your life and makes you who you are. And it's all okay. Do you know what part of your current mindset was cultivated on your own or by others? Is the mindset you have right now serving you? Childhood experiences account for much of who we become as adults. Sometimes you don't realize the impact,

either the good or the bad, until you've lived some years. Love yourself unconditionally, and know that your life matters and you've got everything you need inside to get where you want to go.

2. Recognize your superpowers. What are the areas where you excel or make the most impact? When do you feel most alive by being you? Fulfillment comes when we find our strengths for ourselves, live into them, and let others feel them. Your superpowers will naturally reveal themselves in every area of your life if you let them—career, hobbies, travel, friendships, everything.

3. If you know you need a reshape and you don't know where to start, inspiration can come from others who are excelling where you would like to go. If you make yourself open to it, other people's stories give some of the best education life can bring. Find a mentor, take a class, learn a new skill, ask lots of questions, be inquisitive. You might be surprised how other people are willing to give advice when they see you working on your dream.

CHAPTER 2

THE DREAM JOB THAT PROPELLED ME INTO A WELLNESS RESHAPE

Do the best you can until you know better.
Then when you know better, do better.

MAYA ANGELOU

When the voice on the other end of the line introduced himself as Brian Edwards from William Morris, I didn't need to hear much more. William Morris Talent Agency, now WME, represents some of the biggest names in the entertainment business. I couldn't believe I was even on the phone with them. Brian was from Covington, Louisiana, a couple of hours away from my hometown of Breaux Bridge, and little did I know, a huge pageant fan. He said, "Our Miss Louisiana is now Miss USA; as soon as you took that stage at the Miss USA pageant, I knew you would win the crown! I am bringing you in and getting you signed!" At the time Brian was the executive assistant to Betty Fanning, one of the top commercial agents at William Morris, a legend in her own right, handling talent for soap operas and commercials. True to his word, Brian brought me in and, sure enough, he signed me to the agency. He turned out to be my angel. Little did I know how influential he'd be throughout my life.

Within a month, everything started falling into place. The first five auditions that I went out on, I ended up booking—beginning with a role on NBC's top-rated daytime soap opera, *Sunset Beach*. Brian wasted no time promoting my "debut" and arranged for the *Los Angeles Times* to do a full-page feature story with a reporter covering me on set. Other roles followed, including one for the daytime soap opera *The Young and the Restless*. I'd grown up watching all the CBS daytime soaps, so this was very exciting for me. On Fridays, when all my aunts came to spend the day at my grandmother's after getting their hair done by my mom, we'd all watch *The Price Is Right* together, followed by the lineup of CBS's soap operas.

I knew all the players and all their storylines; I felt like they were my own family. So, at CBS's studios, I walked the hallways, seeing the soundstages where my favorite shows were shooting. I saw props from *The Price Is Right*, like the big wheel. I saw the names of the stars of my favorite daytime actors on the dressing room doors. I nearly had to pinch myself to prove I wasn't dreaming. This was unbelievable. I looked up and saw Jeanne Cooper, the actress who played the formidable Katherine Chancellor on *The Young and the Restless* for years. Before I knew it I yelled across the hallway, "Katherine! Hi! It's so nice to see you!" I called her by her character's name, I was so excited and starstruck. She was probably thinking, *Oh my gosh, who is this child? Who let her in the building?*

I was then ushered into the casting office for my audition, and I booked the job. I honestly don't know how I kept landing these roles, one right after the other. I was the new girl on the block, and quite frankly, I didn't know what in the heck I was doing. I didn't even know that I didn't have to memorize the lines; you could just read off the pages. Brian gave me some very simple advice that still works today: show up on time, be prepared, be your best, and everything else will fall into place. And trust me, I was always prepared and went into each new opportunity mentally and physically present. I noticed that after each of my auditions, the casting agents would look at each other as if to say, *We may have something here.* Brian would promptly call me with the positive feedback he received, and that really boosted my confidence in a business I was so new in. I was so excited when I told my family. They couldn't wait to look for me on their favorite soaps! But it wasn't long before Brian sent me out for an audition that changed everything for me.

"This is Doritos, Ali! It's a national commercial," he said on the phone. "This is a big deal." But it was raining, and I was worried about driving down the streets of Los Angeles in my brand-new white Trans Am, part of my prize package from Miss USA, with my *Thomas Guide to LA and Orange County* on the seat beside me. (My friends to this day tease me about driving that car, but I was just thrilled to *have* a car, a convertible at that, in California. This was my idea of the California dream, straight out of an episode of *Beverly Hills 90210*.) I made every excuse in the book not to go. But Brian wouldn't give up. He called back and said, "Ali, they have been casting for the past two months and really want to bring you in for the producers call, which means they were not 100 percent sold on the finalists chosen for the call-backs. This is a good sign and could turn out very well for you! So don't start with me, Missy, you really need to go in!"

So I went. I'll never forget seeing the beautiful women in chairs lined against the wall, waiting their turn to go in. I walked over to read the storyboard. It showed that "the girl" was supposed to dance around and pretend to be catching a Doritos chip with her mouth. I thought, *Oh, gosh, should I just leave? Do I really want to do this today?* But then, *What's the harm in trying?* I surrendered to the opportunity.

In that moment before I was called in to meet with the ad agency executives, casting director, and producers, I realized I needed to shift my mindset. I quickly flipped the switch on my thinking. I thought, *Okay. This is an awesome opportunity. I am here, so let's kill this audition.* Then I wondered, *How can I set myself apart? What can I do to be different that they haven't seen before—something uniquely me?*

All In

That question was critical. Because truly the most important thing any of us can do, whether it's at work or in parenting or being a friend or spouse, is to be true to who we are. Acting is about letting your authentic self come through while you're acting out the words someone else has written. It's catching their vision and living it out. I just needed to draw on who I was in this wild scenario they'd dreamed up.

Growing up I'd spent years in dance and gymnastic classes and cheerleading. I learned this really cool front handspring where I'd land in a pike. It was kind of a party trick, and I knew I could do it in a small space. I could also do a cartwheel where I'd land by flipping my leg up and go into a split. I thought, *Well, I can do that too.* When they called my name to come in, I went into the audition room where this James Bond music was playing. I did those two tricks and I turned to catch the chip. That was it. By the time I got to my car, about fifteen minutes later, Brian called to say I had booked the job.

On the last day of filming the commercial at the Universal Studios lot, the Doritos executives told us that this was going to be a major commercial campaign. Everyone on the set was ecstatic. I knew that was an important thing in itself, but I did not realize how big of a deal this actually was until Brian called me weeks later and said the commercial was going to premiere during the upcoming Super Bowl in January 1998, adding that he had booked me as a guest on the late-night talk show *Sinbad* for Monday after the game to promote the product. The Frito-Lay team was confident that the spot would end up being the number one Super Bowl commercial that year. And they were right.

I didn't realize that to air a thirty-second spot cost more than a million dollars during the Super Bowl, the most-watched live event on television with almost 100 million people tuning in, many caring as much about the ads as the game itself. Honestly, I was just glad to have the job. All I knew is that I left the set that day satisfied with the work I'd put in. I didn't really think about it again until I was at Super Bowl XXXII in San Diego with my then-boyfriend, a football player.

The game was on a movie-theater-size screen, and I remember seeing myself on this big screen for the first time. I felt like I was melting down into my chair. Thankfully no one had recognized it was me yet. But there I was in living color, flipping in the air, landing into splits to catch a Dorito in my mouth. I didn't know whether to cheer or hide! Not until I heard the entire crowd around me burst into applause and cheers did I take a sigh of relief. I realized in that moment that I was living out one of my dreams.

By this time, Brian Edwards and I were roommates. Even in Los Angeles we Louisianians stick together. I will never forget what he told me after that commercial aired. "Get ready, girl. Your life is about to change." And he was right.

The day after the Super Bowl, the front page of the *New York Post* proclaimed, "A Star Is Born During Super Bowl XXXII." My wonderful manager Elissa Leeds called to say that the phone had been ringing off the hook. (Elissa and I have been together for more than twenty-five years now.) People were calling her with offers for me—for a record deal (evidently it didn't matter that I can't sing), appearances on TV shows, movie opportunities, even dates with high-profile celebrities! It was pretty insane. My career took off in ways I never could have imagined. I felt like I'd finally arrived in this crazy town, and it had happened so fast. But everything was about to change again.

Because I'd grown up in small-town Louisiana where courteous drivers take their time and the busiest roads are slow compared to the LA highways, it took some time for me to adjust to driving in LA. So maybe it's no surprise that on my way to shoot a few episodes of a show I was guest starring in, a show called *Pensacola Wings of Gold*, I was in a car accident that left me literally and proverbially shaken. After the collision, my first thought was how grateful I was to have survived. The damage to my car was pretty bad. Medics checked me out and said I didn't need to be hospitalized. Little did I know then that the residual effects of that tremendous impact would haunt me for decades. My neck, back, and shoulders were never the same afterward. Sleep became an issue because I had trouble getting comfortable. The dull, aching pain would show up almost every night. During the days, sometimes without any warning, my shoulder burned like it was being pierced with a hot knife. But I was working nonstop and living the life of my dreams. I wasn't going to complain, and who would listen if I did?

The Doritos commercial had catapulted me into the next level as an actress, and I worked for ten more years without a break until I had my first child, Estela, because I loved the work so much.

Create a Life You Love

When I married my husband, Alejandro, and we started our family, I began looking for ways to accommodate family life. My mom had done it so beautifully, always caring for us while staying productive and fulfilled. Since she had a salon next to our home, she was always there for us close by, and she still kept up with all her passion projects. I was determined to do the same—to find a way to be there for my family and stay productive and fulfilled in my career. But I often felt torn. When I was working, I felt guilt about being away from family. There had to be a better balance.

I felt like I'd found my dream job when I landed a job on *Hollywood Today Live*—a steady role on a daily talk show syndicated around the country. I'd always enjoyed talk TV. I love people, and I'm naturally curious—after all, I am from southwest Louisiana; I can talk to a tree if I need to. This job seemed like the perfect fit. I visualized this new career move as being great for my family. How much better could it get?

The reality was less than ideal. I'd be up at 5:00 a.m.—which felt like the middle of the night for me because of my chronic back and shoulder pain. I normally tossed and turned most of the night, finally falling asleep at 4:00 a.m. I was in by 6:00 for hair and makeup and research, then we'd go live at 9:00 a.m. Now, I'd done plenty of live TV work before this. I knew that when you're live, you have to have all cylinders firing. It's a challenge. I wasn't by myself reading off a prompter and then tossing it to a package. I was with three other people who were all at the top of their game.

Rude Awakening

I had wanted to do a talk show for years, and this dream job was a panel show where I'd get to work alongside amazing hosts Ross Mathews, Garcelle Beauvais, Amanda Salas, Tanner Thomason, and a rotating seat of guest hosts each week. I imagined this job would be perfect, with a call time at 6:00 a.m., straight into hair and makeup, meeting with producers to prep for the show and guests, in at 8:15 a.m., live at 9:00 a.m., and done by 10:00 a.m. An ideal schedule. I'd pictured getting in a workout, grabbing groceries for dinner, working until it was time to pick up the kids from school, running them around to their afternoon activities, cooking a nice dinner, and finally ending the night with a glass of wine while catching up with my husband. Sounds great and totally doable, right?

Unfortunately, it didn't play out like that.

The reality was that I found myself absolutely exhausted. I could barely function. In the middle of filming, when I was about to interject a comment to contribute to the conversation, I'd find myself thinking one thing and then it would come out of my mouth a completely different way. Or worse, I'd lose my train of thought altogether. This was *live* television, so when the producer counted down, it was time to be on your A game. Taking a few moments to search for the right words was not an option. Because I was the new kid on the block at *Hollywood Today Live*, I began to think that I could possibly lose the job I'd prayed for.

I've always loved a challenge, and I love to perform. But I was not performing well. I was on live TV, listening to the guest talk, nodding and thinking of something to say and then, *ugh*, what came out of my mouth would hit completely differently than I'd planned. It was so frustrating. At first, I thought, *It's just early. I need more coffee or food.* My brain felt foggy. I needed to snap out of this if I was going to keep this job.

My frustration didn't end there. Coming off the adrenaline of a live show and having worked myself to a frenzy to prep the night before, I was in no shape to work out after we wrapped. I'd arrive home from work around noon and, instead of slipping into work-out gear, I'd slide back into my PJs. I'd snack on chips or brownies (because that's what I was craving), then close my eyes and sleep right up until it was time to pick up the kids from school.

Meanwhile, issues I'd been pushing to the side, thinking they would pass, started to pile up. I felt off, but, I wasn't "sick" enough to go to the doctor. Have you ever had that feeling? I had poor digestion, maybe going to the bathroom once or twice a week if I was lucky. My mother pointed out that my hair part was getting wider—in other words, I was losing hair. I had low sex drive, constant fatigue, mood swings, anxiety, poor sleep, mild depression—the list went on. In the past I'd pushed through feeling poorly. But somehow this was different. I couldn't pretend I was okay anymore.

Refusing to Settle

I decided to admit what was really going on in my life and my body. I turned to my girlfriends—friends I've been close with since before kindergarten and who knew me well. When I finally acknowledged what was going on and asked if they were going through any of the same things, one said, "Oh Ali, that's what happens when we age."

"These things are inevitable," another said. "After all, we're over forty."

I was stunned. They were passing all these things off as aging—as if feeling miserable was predestined, unavoidable.

Something in me resisted, hard. I wasn't going to let my friends or myself throw in the towel. I wanted so much more for us. I said, "Oh, no! It's not going to go down like this. I want to live a vibrant life. I'm willing to fight for it! I am going to fight for every hair on my head. I am going to fight for making love and actually wanting to. I am going to fight for good-quality sleep. I am going to fight for the energy to run around with my kids, laughing and playing with them instead of sitting on the sidelines of my life. This isn't working for me, so I'm going to change it. I am going to reshape this area of my life because I am worth it!"

Taking Charge of My Health

It was time to question some of the assumptions I'd been making about my health. I recognized that I needed to treat my body and health in a different way than before. I had to get to the root of the issues I was having, not just look at the symptoms and prescribe something to make them go away. I needed to get to the bottom of it. Could any of the issues be related? What was really going on here? I did not want to feel this way anymore, and I was committed to doing the work. I instinctively felt that if I knew what was going on in my body, I could take positive action.

There had to be something I could do to take back my health. So I went to see a naturopathic doctor. Never before had a doctor taken such an extensive history with me—it was almost like a therapy session. She asked questions I had never been asked by a traditional doctor. Most doctors take about fifteen minutes to get a patient's health history before making a diagnosis. Not her. She took the time to really get to know my history and hear me out. We talked for at least an hour. It was so refreshing to feel heard and seen. She let me know that while what I was experiencing might be "normal" in the sense that lots of people experience those symptoms, what I was experiencing wasn't optimal. And it wasn't necessary. She encouraged me to listen to what my body was telling me.

After that she did some bloodwork to get a baseline read and understand what was going on with my health. When we went through the results of my bloodwork together, it was like drinking from a firehose. There was so much new information! She taught me things I'd never really thought to ask about before. She showed me how stress impacts the immune system, and how things like toxins, sugar, food allergies, gut health, hormones, diet, exercise, and sleep affect the way I was feeling and performing, mentally and physically.

She didn't just look at my symptoms and name them with a "disease" (literally, a dis-ease), she helped me see that my body is complex and beautifully synchronized. She taught me about the systems of my body working together. I vaguely remembered learning about these systems in school, but until that moment I'd taken for granted the way I walked through this life. My mindset, my environment and surroundings, what I was putting on and in my body, my relationships, my daily practices like prayer and meditation, my sleep—all were affecting my health and my sense of well-being. I hadn't considered that they might need regular care and attention.

Around that same time, Tony Robbins and his beautiful wife, Sage, who are producers on one of my husband's films, were so kind to invite Alejandro and me to his Unleash the Power Within event in Los Angeles. Listening to Tony's message, seeing the energy he had at sixty years old, jumping on the stage, running through the audience, I thought to myself, *I want that! I want to feel that way!* That pushed me over the edge to take control. He also said something that weekend that has really stuck with me, and I'll repeat it: Everything I wanted was on the other side of fear. We'll talk more about that later. But during those few days with Tony, a fire was lit inside of me to look at my life as a whole, to identify those areas that were not serving me, starting with my health because that was so pressing at the time.

I also heard from Dave Asprey at that event, the father of biohacking and founder of Bulletproof. He spoke about mitochondria, I was so perplexed by this. Why did he think this was so important? After all, he was speaking to thousands of people that weekend, so he must have thought there was something special about these parts of our cells, which are often called the "powerhouses" of each cell in our bodies. I had never thought about my health from a cellular level. Before I started my reshape journey, I thought about working out to be healthy or eating better to be healthy. When I felt unhealthy or sick, I went to the doctor and got a prescription and got better after a while, but it seemed like that was happening pretty often. But, again, I'd never thought about taking control of my health, understanding my body and how it functions, and possibly "hacking" my biology. I hadn't thought about mitochondrial dysfunction, and maybe that was why I had no energy and my body and mind were aging. I was thirsty for knowledge, determined to ask questions and to learn. I was ready to look at my life in a completely different way and do whatever I needed to do to feel better.

Empowered to Thrive

My naturopathic doctor showed me how the body constantly prioritizes its needs. That made me feel so grateful! The human body really is pretty amazing. My eyes were opened to its possibilities, and I was energized to give my body what it needed. I didn't want to just get back to normal. I wanted to find a way to thrive like never before. I knew it was possible.

But all my issues didn't just disappear with this new information. I had lots of work to do.

The main areas I focused on initially were:

- Diet. I started keeping a food diary to be more mindful of how my body reacted to what I was eating. I began increasing my water intake. And I began eliminating sugar and processed foods and adding in more vegetables and healthy fats. I started to look at the source of where my food came from.
- Switching my morning coffee routine. I had gotten used to using products that were laden with chemicals every day for years.
- Fasting. I implemented intermittent fasting a few days a week.
- Vitamins. I started taking specific supplements based on what my bloodwork showed, providing what my body actually needed instead of what I thought I needed.
- Cleansing. I did a doctor-observed candida cleanse to get my microbiome in balance. During that process I fully broke out in hives on my face, neck, and chest as my body was ridding itself

of toxins. Ross Mathews, my friend and cohost on *Hollywood Today*, whom I adore, made such fun of me, calling me the "sickest healthy person he knew." He also did a "hive watch" on the show, checking in daily on how I was doing. We had to announce it because there was no hiding it.

- Lowering inflammation. We did this with diet and supplements to help with the chronic pain issues that I had been dealing with for more than twenty years.
- Sleep. My sleep habits had gotten worse over the years. I took the first step by not exposing myself to any blue light from my phone or computer screen an hour before bed.
- Eliminating toxins and allergens from my home and kitchen.
- Addressing adrenal fatigue due to stress with supplements.
- Using clean products on my skin.
- Setting aside a half hour every morning to mindfully meditate and pray.

These new life changes resulted in immediate benefits that grew with time. I could tell right away that I had more energy. I realized it is possible to heal and promote good health from within, at a cellular level. This was incredible to me. What a game changer! Thank you, Dave Asprey! I wanted to learn more, know more, and take back my health. I was going to become a *wellness explorer*. I was on fire with excitement and I wanted to share this not only with my girlfriends in Louisiana but also with every woman who might be feeling the same way.

It was a turning point. I was on a quest to seek out top doctors, researchers, scientists, innovators, and spiritual advisers—asking questions many women want answered but don't know how or who to ask.

With the guidance of my naturopathic doctor, I listened to my body and learned tangible next steps that I could take to change things. I no longer felt helpless. I could see a way forward. I didn't change everything overnight. I started with only a few of the above at first—after all, this way of living was all new to me. Gradually I was able to incorporate all these actions throughout that first year of my health journey.

Part of me worried that I'd slide back into feeling poorly. I wanted lasting change. Extreme makeovers overnight are likely to come undone. So instead of going cold turkey—like giving up coffee (only because of what I was putting in it), which would be impossible—I began to gradually upgrade my routines.

I felt so empowered after having tried some of these things and seeing benefits. I was fired up. I was going to reshape my health—and become stronger and healthier than ever. It is 100 percent a choice; I had to choose me. It's the things we do every day that make the biggest difference.

Coffee Recipes

I have two favorite day-starters: my indulgent, yummy Supergirl coffee and my Let's Get Lean "Game On" coffee, the one I do when I am intermittent fasting or being really on top of my diet.

SUPERGIRL COFFEE

I make this on most weekends and during the week when I feel like I am going to treat myself.

Ingredients

8 oz organic coffee (it matters), brewed
Lakanto Monkfruit sweetener to liking

1 scoop Laird Hamilton Superfood Creamer
1 scoop Primal Kitchen Vanilla Collagen Creamer
Dash of pumpkin spice
Dash of cocoa powder
1 to 2 tablespoons Bulletproof Brain Octane C8 MCT Oil

Method

Blend in a blender for extra frothiness. I serve in my Yeti to keep it hot until almost noon. I also drink out of a stainless steel straw so the coffee won't touch my teeth much in order to prevent staining.

"GAME ON" COFFEE

Ingredients

One cup well-made black coffee
1 to 2 tablespoons Bulletproof Brain Octane C8 MCT Oil

Method

We are very picky about our coffee and how we prepare it. My husband has beans roasted only a few days before they are delivered, and he grinds them as we need them each morning. He finds the perfect grind size at the perfect temp and pours over a very specific way for the exact time to get the best cup of coffee he can make. You might think it is a bit much, and if I told you that he traveled with all his coffee gear, you would think he is crazy. I thought so too at first. But I never thought I could drink coffee black until I had it this way. It was a complete and total game changer. Also, the ritual and ceremony of making coffee this way in the morning is a meditation in itself.

To make "Game On" coffee, I pour some of this delicious coffee, black, into my Vitamix blender (after I've preheated it with hot water, then transferred that hot water to my Yeti to warm it too, dumping it out after it's warm). I add a tablespoon or two of Bulletproof Brain Octane C8 MCT Oil to round out that delicious coffee, making it a creamier version of itself, and *voilà*!

Elevated Health

Everything that was off in my life had been connected, so as I began to adjust and make improvements, it all elevated. It all lifted. It was all connected.

My thinking was clearer. My hair started to thicken, and my nails grew harder more quickly. (This took the longest.) My digestion improved. For the first time in my life, I was eliminating daily without the help of laxatives. (Insert fireworks here!) I began to exercise smarter, which releases endorphins, serotonin, and dopamine, which led to feeling even better. My sex drive improved. I no longer was experiencing that afternoon slump. My mood improved.

Everything felt a little bit better! To sum it up, I was no longer sitting on the sidelines of my life. I was in the game and I was ready to play.

Contagious Enthusiasm

The difference between how I'd been feeling and how I now felt was nothing short of miraculous. I had more energy and fewer symptoms. Now that I knew about this next level of health, I was just itching to share it with everyone who'd listen. I told my girlfriends, and they

were hopeful. Some began to
experiment with the methods I'd
implemented, applying them to
their unique situations, and they
saw results too. I am not saying
that all was well immediately. It
was and still is a journey for each
one of us. Your journey may be
different. Your process to get your

> I don't care how old
> I am. I am going to
> the bouncy house.
>
> *Doug The Pug*
> *on Twitter*

reshape may be different, but these were the steps that worked for me.
I hope they can inspire you.

A Fire Is Lit

So that's how wellness became such a passion for me. I could spend a
lifetime just catching up to the science of it all. And the data is growing by the second. There's so much to learn! After working with my
naturopathic doctor, I was feeling so much better, but I still needed
fine-tuning. I needed to seek out experts. I was now building my
wellness team. I got connected with some incredible minds who were
moving the needle in their specific fields. It started when I cornered
Dr. Michael Breus, "The Sleep Doctor," while we were both guests on
a talk show. I was more concerned with connecting with him than
I was about my segment that was coming up. I begged him for help
with my sleep, and we began a friendship. He has played a big part in
my sleep and my pain journey as well. Remember, it's all connected.

Of course by then I knew Tony Robbins, basically the world's
life coach, and Dave Asprey of Bulletproof and *The Human Upgrade*
podcast, who is on a lifelong quest to enhance the human body's
functionality. I also connected with Robin Sharma, author of *The*

Monk Who Sold His Ferrari, and Naomi Whittel of *Glow15* and *High Fiber Keto*. Then there was Jim Kwik, the world's number one brain coach, and the list goes on and on. Each conversation, each book I read, each podcast I listened to stoked my passion for this subject.

These expert researchers and scientists in the health and wellness world were teaching me that it is absolutely possible to turn back your biological clock. We can now do things that can make us ten and twenty years younger and more powerful than ever. They each brought a wealth of knowledge and insight. These conversations fueled my passion to learn more.

My curiosity energized me. And once I dug in, I started to see results pretty quickly. I was reshaping my life in profound ways. It was thrilling! As a natural-born sharer, I could not keep all of the life-changing information to myself. After getting my girlfriends from Louisiana onboard, I also started to share on air what was happening. Many women responded with questions and encouragement. I realized then how many women could benefit from the solutions that were working for me personally. It was so exciting! I might not have a medical degree or deep training, but I had access to the people who did. I could share what I was learning from these authorities, sharing as a friend. I wanted to help as many women as I could.

So my business partner Rebekah Hubbell and I launched RE/SHAPE, a lifestyle company to serve women around the world with the curated resources that are integral for a full-life reshape—heart, mind, soul, and health. I wanted to take what I have learned and share it with women who are in the same place I was.

To do that, I engage with amazing experts and interview them to share their systems, routines, and education, with our RE/SHAPE community. I partner with companies I truly believe in. If their products have improved my life or are game changers for me, they become a hero product with RE/SHAPE. We provide extensive content daily across multiple platforms that can be applied in your life as you step into your own reshape. The foundation for a complete reshape is gathered there, with the resources, tools, and support system you need to achieve your goals. RE/SHAPE was created just for you.

I used to feel like I was sitting on the sidelines of my life, but compared to how I feel now, I know it's all been worth it. Looking back, I realize that part of my resolve to reshape my health and not let it dictate my future came from previous life experience. I'd been knocked to my knees in the past in very different ways—*forced reshapes*, as I like to call them. I'd lived through it and come out stronger. I knew I could do it again. And that's a story in and of itself.

———————— RESHAPE WRAP-UP ————————

What is your mindset about health? Are you an active participant in your overall wellness? Or are you the way I was, where you often look past those nagging issues that slow you down and put more strain on your daily life?

Have you ever viewed your overall health and lifestyle vitality from a holistic perspective? This way of thinking has completely transformed how I walk through my life. It was a game changer for me to partner with a medical adviser who could offer comprehensive testing, explain the results, and offer options that would help me. It allowed me to experience the next level of health I never thought possible.

It comes down to a lifestyle evaluation and figuring out the patterns you need to reshape to create a life you love. Patterns, habits, and certain mindsets can get in the way of living a vibrant life. Developing a proactive mindset in all areas of your life will allow you to flourish as you were intended to. We all settle into life sometimes, often without realizing it. But I am here to remind you not to settle—

that you are worth it. I will help you fight for a thriving life. We can all do better together.

RESHAPE MOVES ——————————————

1. Listen to what your body is telling you. Don't wait to figure it out. Become your own health advocate. You are worth more than waiting until you crash to take care of yourself.
2. Medicating symptoms is not the answer long term. Get to the root of the issue as quickly as you can. Do the work to find the resources and tools you need to reshape the areas of your health that are not serving you.
3. Finding a like-minded community is a blessing beyond words. Trading health hacks, recipes, doctor referrals, and creating basic accountability will immediately level up your mindset and create a healthy environment you can thrive in.

CHAPTER 3

RESHAPE YOUR FOOD

Eating for Vitality from a

Self-Declared Foodie

The things that excite us aren't random.
They're connected to our unique purpose.

TERRIE DAVOLL HUDSON

Anyone who knows me knows that I have always been passionate about food. I can remember as a child getting so excited when I would find out what my mom was making for dinner. Whether it was crawfish étouffée or a gumbo, I was ready to savor it completely and always went back for seconds. Oh, and the cakes my aunts would make from scratch. Like the pineapple upside-down cake or my grandmother's *gâteau sec* cookies—a hundred-year-old recipe that brings me to tears because they are so good. To this day, when my Aunt Vicky makes them for me for Christmas, I hide the entire bowl of those cookies so I can have them all to myself. I have never been one of those girls who would shy away from food. I always say, "I don't completely trust a woman who doesn't eat."

As I have gotten older and have expanded my palate, I have learned so much about nutrition and how what I put into my body directly affects how I feel. It affects my energy, my digestion, my sleep, my emotions—everything. Discovering this changed everything. How could I go back to my old habits after that? It was as if I was seeing the world in a whole new way. I was eager to learn more.

Rice and Gravy

I grew up with very little nutritional knowledge. I don't think I even remember having a salad or many vegetables on the dinner table, and if we did have them, I wasn't eating them. But, *again*, I've always enjoyed good food.

Enjoying great food and the experience around the table makes me feel more alive, in more ways than one. I get so much joy from the tastes, smells, and the visual aesthetic of beautifully prepared food. Plus, food is literally energy—fuel for the building blocks of our bodies. When I'm eating, I'm nurturing my body. On some level I've known that instinctually all my life, even when I had virtually no understanding of nutrition.

As a kid I loved food because it represented family and culture. It was a way to celebrate and share traditions, not to mention that it was delicious. My grandmothers were both excellent cooks, and we gathered for shared meals often. To this day I can recall my Mom Landry's incredible rice and gravy. She marinated her round steak in vinegar all night, which made the most amazing gravy. I could drink it. I'd clean my plate, using my fingernail to scrape up every bit of that delicious dish.

Growing up as I did, it's obvious that starving myself has never been in my DNA. For a brief time before I won Miss Louisiana USA, I had a modeling contract. At five feet, eight inches, I was definitely not tall enough or thin enough by industry standards, but somehow several modeling agencies offered to sign me. I signed with Pauline's, who had offices in Paris, New York, and Miami, and as a result I got to live in all these great places. The idea of it was all so exciting. I'd always dreamed of seeing the world, and this seemed like a good start.

My modeling experience was a revelation to me in many ways. After casting calls, more than once, I got called back to headquarters for a meeting and to get measured. Many conversations ended in, "We think you are great; you just need to lose a few pounds if you want to really make it in this business." It was all so vague—and not helpful. They weren't offering me a healthy plan to follow, and I didn't understand how to do what they were asking. While I was eating a bowl of Frosted Flakes cereal every morning, the other models' "breakfast" was smoking a cigarette. Was their not eating a key to success in the runway business? That didn't make sense to me. Maybe my sugary cereal wasn't the best breakfast, but starving myself was not something I was willing to do. Again, I loved food too much. I count myself fortunate to have made it through that time without developing disordered eating issues. The upside was that I finally made the association between weight gain or loss and food. It was a nutritional insight at least.

I soon realized that modeling wasn't something I wanted to continue doing. It wasn't a good fit with who I am and what I bring to the table. So I left it behind and went home to Louisiana to finish college, regroup, and figure out what my next move could be. That's when I thought, *I've got to figure out this job situation.* At the time I was majoring in communications and I was thinking that I would ultimately go into news and, if I was lucky, transition to entertainment television.

Ice Cream Sundaes in First Class

After I got the Doritos commercial campaign, I worked steadily for years in the entertainment business. One of my favorite perks was getting to travel with my dear friend, Davia Matson. She's a makeup artist, hair stylist when needed, wardrobe consultant (because she has the best style), and the one friend who is always completely honest with me. Like me, Davia likes food, but she's definitely not as passionate about it as I am. I'll never forget the first time we were booked to go to New York City together for work, flying first class.

On our long flight they brought us delicious food. Davia is a picker—she eats a little bit of this, a bite of that. She eats everything—nothing is off limits for her—but like I said, she "picks" like a little bird. At the end of that meal on the airplane they brought us an ice cream sundae for dessert. She barely touched hers. When Davia looked over and saw me eyeing her ice cream sundae, she offered it to me and I finished not only mine but every last bit of hers as well! I knew then that we'd be lifelong friends. I've been finishing her food ever since.

On location, I'd always ask locals to find the best, most interesting places to eat. Then I'd get Davia to come along to explore with me. We'd work for hours and get really hungry, then take a cab to these urban gems—sushi, vegetarian, Indian, Chinese, French—you name it, we tried it. These culinary adventures all over the world were expanding my palate and instilling an appreciation around the culinary experience, every nuance of it.

The Accident that Started It All

I've told you that years before my children were born, when I first moved to LA, I was in a car accident that wreaked havoc on my neck and spine. That accident started me down the road of chasing pain, and I would never be the same again. I started getting massages to deal with it. One day the massage therapist asked me about an enlarged place close to my left ear. Up to that point I'd been aware of it, but not really concerned. She said, "You need to see a doctor about this." I was taken aback because she was concerned, so I made an appointment with an ear, nose, and throat specialist. He also looked at it with concern, took some X-rays, and collected a sample of the tissue. He called the next day, saying, "This is a parotid gland tumor. I'm sending you to a specialist at UCLA."

Wait, what? Now *I* was concerned. I'd gone from oblivious to alarmed pretty quickly.

Reshape Bridge

I believe everything in life happens for a reason. If I hadn't been in that car accident, I wouldn't have been getting massages to manage the pain. That means most likely I would not have found that tumor. Those connections never cease to amaze me.

I saw a specialist right away who diagnosed the tumor as benign, thank the Lord, but the rest of the news wasn't very good. That tumor had grown around and engulfed the facial nerve, making its removal complicated. Although my surgeon was one of the best, he warned me that damage or disturbance to the facial nerve during the tumor removal can cause facial paralysis. My surgery was scheduled and I began to fervently pray.

This was another instance where a little bit of self-care—a massage—saved me from what could have been a frightening outcome.

Though the surgery went well, afterward I got a staph infection. So, on top of the pain medications, I had to take antibiotics. While my prognosis was essentially good, it was a lot for my body to process. The anesthesia, pain meds, and antibiotics had me feeling off. I sensed that I needed to reset my body. I checked in for a five-day retreat at the We Care Spa, which specializes in regimens for detoxing the body. Some guests even reported having been cured of "incurable" diseases. At We Care, I was introduced to holistic healing. I learned more about my body in those five days than I ever dreamed possible. I also learned that when you lose your health, you spend your entire life chasing it.

They didn't just treat my body; they taught classes. I learned about nutritional healing, meditation, herbal remedies, essential oils, and all sorts of other natural wonders. For example, on that first spa retreat, I sat in on a breathing class. I didn't understand the hype; after all, I breathe every day I am alive. But I had a lot of time on my hands while I was there, so I thought, *Why not? If anything it will be nice and relaxing.* I had a huge, as Oprah would say, aha moment. I think I took my first full breath of my life in that class. I was taught how to breathe from my lower belly. I immediately went up to the teacher after class and said, "Thank you, thank you, thank you! I didn't know it before, but I've been taking shallow breaths for my whole life. I think I just took my first *real* breaths!"

Digestive Issues

The main goal of my stay at We Care was to flush all the toxins from those medications out of my body. Their cleansing regime was different from anything else I had ever done. You are pretty much fasting from food, with a focus on liquid nutrition, including wheat-grass shots. At that point I was desperate and willing to do anything to feel better.

I also got my first introduction to colonics there. My digestion was really off from all the medicines and needed to be flushed out. It was a humbling experience in many ways. The contents of my intestines were being analyzed by someone I didn't even know. It is amazing

> Breath is the bridge which connects life to consciousness, which unites your body to your thoughts. Whenever your mind becomes scattered, use your breath as the means to take hold of your mind again.
>
> *Thich Nhat Hanh*

what a professional can deduce from what comes out your other end. These people are like archaeologists. They'd talk to me the whole time. I remember one therapist saying, "This one has been there a long time." I was glad to be rid of it, but kind of mortified! They celebrated when I started having bowel movements too. There was no judgment, only a sense that the consequences of what had happened to my body were real, not just in my head. It was liberating. I felt empowered and more in touch with my body than I had in years.

Loopy with Hunger

They helped me to transition back to solid food, but not before I went on a true-blue fast. I'd never fasted before. It was all new to me—and a real awakening to how much I thought about food! One night I went with a few of the other spa guests to see a movie in town. The smell of the popcorn was tantalizing. You have to understand, one of my favorite things in life is to go to the movies and get a big bucket of buttered popcorn and a bag of M&Ms. It used to be Sno-Caps, but they stopped selling those in most movie theaters . . . but that's a whole other story. You get the point: I love the movies and popcorn! During the film, I left my seat to go to the restroom. As I walked, I saw one lone piece of buttered theater popcorn laying there on the carpet. I couldn't take my eyes off it! That little kernel hypnotized me. I was literally thinking of picking it up off the floor and eating it. That sounds crazy, I know, but I was so hungry.

I am happy that I resisted that little piece of popcorn on the floor and surrendered fully to the We Care experience, because this special place in the desert transformed me forever. I now thought about my body, my digestion, my food in a completely different way. I learned how to breathe, how to promote circulation in my body, how to be still. I learned about different modalities to heal my body and spirit.

Nutrition

Becoming a wellness explorer was a turning point. I began to use food to heal my body, and that changed everything for me. I would never be the same. I did it on my own for a while, figuring it out as I went—reading health books, listening to podcasts, going to wellness conventions, and talking to experts. I was introduced to so many food protocols, and they were exciting—methods developed by nutritionists, scientists, and athletes. I pretty much tried them all and saw results with most, but it began to get overwhelming. I knew it was time to bring another team member in. I needed to work with someone who specialized in nutrition and understood the whole body. I needed to be able to share my personal health journey, to share my life, my story. I needed a program that was tailor-made for me, taking into account my pain, sleep, energy, and digestion issues. I needed a coach.

I met Sarah Wragge through Meredith, one of my dear friends from Louisiana. Meredith had been working with Sarah, and I'd seen firsthand how Meredith seemed to glow and radiate health and energy. She looked lean and strong, and I was impressed. Meredith put me in touch with Sarah, and we clicked immediately. I told her everything, just like in a therapy session. She had the same philosophy as me—that you can eat amazing and clean for the majority of the time but you have to live life and indulge every once in a while. You have to be able to drink cocktails and go to great dinners with no guilt, knowing that you will get back at it the following day. Our journey together began.

Meet the Expert: Sarah Wragge

When I met Ali [in April 2019], she was doing a lot of the "right" things: she ate healthy foods and exercised regularly, but she was struggling with *energy* and *digestive issues*—things I hear from new clients daily. During our initial consult, we discussed what her day-to-day life looked like and how we could integrate the Sarah Wragge Wellness Method seamlessly. Ali knew her body well and had been paying attention to what wasn't working well for her, so we were already starting from a good spot. She had a good grasp on the importance of proper nutrition and was eager to learn even more. Ali was ready to reshape her eating habits for the better. Because of that openness and honesty, I was able to quickly home in on the core issues she needed to tackle.

The first thing I told Ali was this: "You don't have to feel bad every day. Together, we can get you back to feeling amazing—likely better than you've ever felt—in just a few weeks." I could say this with confidence because I had been there too. I struggled with digestive and health issues for years, which were exacerbated by working in a high-stress corporate marketing job in New York City. I saw traditional doctor after doctor, but not one could help me get to the root cause of my symptoms. Then, as a last-ditch effort, I worked with a functional medicine practitioner and acupuncturist, which was life changing in so many ways—not only for my personal health but professionally as well.

The SWW Method is about enjoying all life's special moments and delicious food while still feeling your best and most amazing self. I told Ali, there's no deprivation needed; she enjoys eating just as much as I do. My goal is for clients to eat better, not less. It's about honoring your body by giving it what it really wants and needs to have prolonged energy and creating lifestyle change that's truly sustainable.

In Ali's case, I realized we needed to retrain her body to use the right source of fuel for energy. She was eating sugar, and we needed to turn her into a fat burner. We also needed to get her digestive system to work efficiently. To do that, we needed to change how, what, and when she ate.

We started by focusing on four things.

1. Blood-Sugar-Balanced Meals

I worked with Ali to make sure every time she ate, she consumed fiber, protein, and healthy fat, with no added sweeteners. Once we did this, Ali reported back that she was rarely hungry and had fewer cravings.

Another important step was focusing on Ali's morning routine. For years she'd been waking up and consuming loads of coffee spiked with fake creamer and Splenda. This habit was wreaking havoc on her digestive system. Not only was this very acidic, it was chemical-laden, artificial, and sugary, which spiked her blood-sugar levels and set her up for crashes and cravings all day. When she was crashing, she'd reach for more carbs—granola or a bar—and that would perpetuate the sugar-spike cycle. We figured out a way for her to continue to have her morning coffee, but we up-leveled the quality of ingredients she was adding to make sure it was blood-sugar balanced. We added fat, fiber, and protein, which made both of us happy. (You've already seen a few favorite recipes in chapter 2.)

2. Alkalinity

Like a lot of women, Ali's body was very acidic. I was able to teach her some simple things to start balancing out her body's pH naturally. The big improvement for her was when she started drinking a daily green juice—one of my favorite nutrition hacks, since it gives you instant energy without caffeine or sugar. Think of drinking green juice as a nutritional shot to your cells—hydrating, alkalizing, and priming your body for digestion, setting your foundation for the day.

This green-juice habit went a long way toward helping Ali's digestive issues too. When I met her, Ali wasn't going to the bathroom nearly enough. Like many of my clients, she thought it was normal to not go to the bathroom for three or four days. When she started eliminating daily, she was thrilled—and I was too.

In addition to the green juice, I wanted Ali having greens with every meal. This not only helps keep her full but also loads her body with the micronutrients she needs to thrive and continues to support an alkaline state throughout the day. Other ways we increased alkalinity were removing dairy and processed seed oils from her diet and having Ali drink three liters of water daily—the first immediately upon waking to hydrate her body and help flush toxins that were produced overnight.

3. Being Prepared

With Ali's schedule, being prepared was absolutely key. I didn't want her to be in a situation where she'd be stuck choosing between eating something less than optimal, like a bagel, or going hungry. There needed to be good choices at hand that she could quickly grab when she was short on time.

Ali leaned hard into food prep, and that set her up for a successful week ahead. She found she really enjoyed shopping at the farmers' market on weekends, juicing, and doing meal prep to set herself and her family up for the week. That way she made sure they all got nutrient-dense, fiber-rich, protein-packed meals. As she paid more attention to what was going into the meals, she was also able to up-level the quality, seeking out wild fish, organic eggs, and clean ingredients.

4. Meal Timing

One final area we focused on was the timing of Ali's meals. Did you know the average American snacks seventeen times a day? Every time you pick up a bite or take a sip of something—the remainder of your kids' French toast, a handful of almonds, a stick of gum or breath mints—you're engaging the digestive system. By feeding it all the time you're constantly spiking insulin levels and shutting down fat burning. I encouraged Ali to eat three or four times a day—ideally every four hours—and that was it. By giving her body a break between consumption, she was retraining her digestive system and metabolism.

Again, I'm not encouraging anyone to eat less, just less often. When the digestive system isn't constantly engaged, the body learns to burn fat as the primary source of fuel instead of sugar (fruits, carbs). And if you're consuming high-quality foods when you do eat, your body won't crave carbs and sugar for energy.

The goal is what I call "metabolic flexibility," where you can occasionally eat carbs and sugar, but your body goes right back to burning fat instead of craving more carbs and sugar for fuel.

———————

Ali loves to learn, so we were a good team. She started to make empowered, informed choices from day one, which is what I'm all about: empowerment. I teach my clients to have a relationship with food that is friendly, not adversarial. You will never hear me being restrictive about food. Instead, it's about choice. Ali understood that intuitively. She knows we all need those fun indulgences. A perfect example of this is when Ali was traveling, and she and a friend went to a beignet place from their childhood. They ordered the classic beignets—which are fried dough and sugar—and enjoyed every morsel! I said, "Good for you! I love that you're getting to do that!" Because that's what it's all about: feeding your body nutrient-dense, clean food and giving yourself permission to experience the emotions, flavors, textures, and memories that go with eating the occasional "splurge." For me, on Friday nights I choose to have pizza and red wine with my husband, then I'm back at it with my green juice the next morning.

My goal is to get you feeling amazing. Then you can make an informed decision to splurge and pivot right back to your routine. Eating a croissant isn't bad if it's a choice. When you make a choice to eat something that's not optimal for you, instead of going down the shame spiral, you get right back to your usual, healthy ways because you *desire* waking up in the morning feeling great.

What advice would I give readers who want to reshape their eating habits? I'd say you'll see huge change if you do these three things:

When you wake up, drink an entire *liter of water* before having any coffee. Our bodies wake in an acidic state, and it's important to flush out those toxins from yesterday. That will set you up for a healthy start and make you feel good about yourself.

Before coffee, have an *alkaline moment*. Again, I like fresh green juice. My favorite is celery juice, cucumber, lettuce, and ginger, but I'm not picky—any way you can get greens in there is good. If not a green juice, try hot water with half a lemon. Or do a shot of apple cider vinegar or cayenne and lemon juice. It's amazing how much energy you'll have even before coffee! Remember: it helps if you're prepared. Ali makes her celery juice for the week on weekends. If you buy yours in a shop or store, be sure to get pure greens—no fruit juice or sugar added.

Finally, make your first meal of the day a *blood-sugar-balancing* choice. Think: *protein + fat + fiber*. Too many people start their day with carbs, spiking their blood-sugar levels and setting themselves up to crash and crave all day long. Instead I recommend eggs and spinach with avocado; chia pudding with organic almond butter; or (my favorite) a smoothie made from spinach, nut butter, and collagen powder. I especially like liquid nutrition as a start (or end) to a day because the body doesn't have to work so hard to extract the nutrients—it's easily accessible energy without the crash.

By making these three good choices at the start of your day, you'll start to feel more energy and better digestion, like Ali did. And feeling great is what it's all about!

Eating well was really the key to feeling amazing. That discovery was literally a lifetime in the making. I had tapped into something that had always been important to me: my love for good food.

Now that I fully understood the effects of healthy eating choices, it became so clear to me that being a food lover is a superpower, not a flaw. Food isn't the enemy. Food is magic! Eating *less* isn't the goal. Eating *best* is. To live my best life, eating well is key.

Conscious Eating

To respect my body, I respect the food I'm putting into it.

I'd shifted my focus from what *tasted* good to what *was* good. That means eating lots of vegetables, healthy fats, fiber, and clean proteins. Don't get me wrong: on special occasions or when I'm at a party, I indulge with zero guilt. My daily mindset, however, is eating clean and healthy foods. Drinking lots of water and teas daily is key too, as is enjoying healthy carbs in the evening.

I started to eat at home more, to prepare and cook for myself and my family. I never want to settle for less with the taste of my food. I'd grown up in a place known for its delicious cuisine, after all, so I started to experiment with taking some of my favorite dishes and making them healthy. Before that I'd used a meal-delivery service because I was working so much. It was convenient and such a luxury, but I gave it up because I wanted to learn about what foods and portions are good for my body. I'd been letting someone else determine that. I wanted to take ownership and learn for myself, if this reshape was going to stick. I fell in love with vegetables and ways to prepare them that would not skimp on taste. It was meditative for me, putting so much care finding the perfectly sourced ingredients and preparing them with love for me and my family. It was as satisfying as the meal itself. I felt good knowing the ingredients that went into what we were eating.

These days I don't think of preparing food as a chore I can hire out; it's a pleasure and a privilege. I enjoy finding healthy ingredients and discovering new recipes.

When I picked my writing partner up at the airport for the

writing retreat to map out this book, my trunk was so full of groceries we could hardly fit her suitcase in. I'd brought overnight oats,
colorful veggies, two kinds of hummus, nuts, grain-free crackers,
homemade green juice, coffee, my favorite creamer and sweetener,
tea, and plenty of water. Honestly, there would have been much
more, but I planned for us to try out area restaurants for our meals!

Shopping for fresh, healthy foods can be fun and exciting. You
should see how excited I get in a Whole Foods! When I get home,
I immediately prep all the food I need for the week, chopping fresh
vegetables and fruits. Then I'm ready to cook for myself and my family and friends. Food brings me more joy than ever!

Most of all, I am a conscious eater, mindful of what *and* when
I eat. Consciously eating means listening to hunger cues and being
aware of the eating experience, not zoning out or eating to go numb.
I also pay attention to how my body reacts to what I consume. Do I
feel gassy? Bloated? Constipated? Sleepy and lethargic? Or do I feel
pleasantly satiated? Energized? Invigorated? Paying attention helps
me make those little tweaks to go from good to great. I've learned to
really listen to my body. If I'm hungry, I eat something. If I need red
meat around the time of my cycle, I'll eat it. If I'm tired, I take a nap. I
try to do all this mindfully. The more I tune in and listen to what my
body is telling me, the more clarity I have around my cravings and
what my body needs.

Checking In

I don't wait until summer swimsuit time or a New Year's resolution
to check in with my body. Once a month or every three months I like
to do a refresh, like intermittent fasting, cutting my late-night snacks,
upping my water intake, getting on track with my morning digestive

routine, having bone broth or a veggie purée soup for dinner. Starting my day with a healthy protocol sets me up for success for the rest of the day. When I choose to have a blueberry scone on Sunday morning with my coffee, I notice that the rest of the day I am more likely to take a few fries from the kids, munch on a bag of chips, and things like that. This is such a great way for me to be continually checking in, reevaluating, fine-tuning not just my diet but also my life.

Autophagy

Recently I decided I needed another reset but didn't want to leave my husband and children for five days. That's when I discovered water fasting. No spa or retreat needed! Just me and my gallon water bottle.

I learned about fasting from Naomi Whittel, wellness explorer, CEO, and author of *Glow15*. Naomi grew up on an organic biodynamic farm. Her chemist father taught her the elements of a health-promoting diet, which you'd think was all she'd ever need to know. But as an adult she suffered from debilitating eczema. Nothing seemed to help. For a time she was helped by herbs and acupuncture, but when she was pregnant, she realized the herbs she'd been ingesting were causing a dangerous toxicity. This experience empowered her on a journey to maximize her health and vitality. Naomi's Facebook group is where I learned about fasting to promote autophagy.

What is autophagy? Well, "auto" means "self" and "phage" means "eat." I began to see how autophagy is actually marvelous. See, when the body isn't busy processing food, the autophagy process is triggered, creating an orderly removal of unnecessary or dysfunctional cells. It's a house cleaning at the cellular level. A reshape! The stressed, toxified cells in the body get swept out to make way for healthier, new cells.

When I read about this, I thought it made total sense. I said, "I'm going to try this tomorrow!" I can be a bit spontaneous about these things sometimes, but I felt like I was called to do this in that moment.

Alejandro was in Colombia for a very important film project, *Sound of Freedom*, about the lifesaving work of Tim Ballard. Alejandro shared with me that the funding hadn't all come in yet and they were about to start shooting. As I was researching how to do a water fast, I discovered that some people fast with an intention and prayer. When hunger pangs hit, you can focus on that intention. This gives the mind a precision and focus. How wonderful: wellness exploration with added mindset determination!

The core message of the film is against child trafficking, so I felt like I could honor that with my fast. What was so wild was that on day two of my fast, a colleague of Naomi's, Dr. Daniel Pompa, posted videos talking viewers through each day of the fast and what to expect. I watched and was stunned when Dr. Pompa mentioned Tim Ballard—the subject of my husband's film! I was speechless. What are the chances that I decided to do this fast after hearing about it for the first time on Naomi's Facebook post, then thought that I should fast for a cause—the complete financing of the movie *Sound of Freedom* about real-life hero Tim Ballard, who was saving children's lives all over the world from trafficking—only to be listening in on the daily instructions of the fast from Dr. Daniel Pompa, who then mentioned Tim Ballard's name on day two? I called Alejandro and then Tim to encourage them and let them know I was fasting with the intention and prayer for funding of the film. On the fifth and last day of my fast, the money came together.

It would be hard to scientifically connect fasting with funding, but I know that water fasting caused a biological reset in me, as do many other types of fasting. Here are just a few of the potential benefits:

- improved blood sugar control
- reduction of inflammation
- decreased blood pressure levels
- boost in brain function
- weight loss
- increase in human growth hormone (HGH) secretion
- autophagy

Why do I do these sorts of things? I'm naturally curious. New information excites me. I don't mind taking risks. I'm happy to be the guinea pig to test the ropes to see what will happen. If there are benefits, it invigorates me even more to share them with you!

Hydration

Are you drinking enough water? Hydration is absolutely essential for good health. Side effects from not drinking enough water include headaches, constipation, dry or chapped lips, increased wrinkles, low urine output, dizziness, and lightheadedness.

When my kids were younger, I made hydration a game with them. After they urinated I'd have them check to see if the urine was clear or yellow. For them, it was fun—a sort of surprise. Clear means you're fully hydrated; yellow means the body needs more water.

Think of it this way: water is literally life-giving. Drinking enough water helps us experience good digestion, elastic skin, even clear thinking. It's essential for good health in mind, body, and spirit! I typically get down three and a half liters daily, but my goal is always a gallon.

Tip: I have water with me at all times. I have done this for years. My preference is to put my entire day's water in one jug so I can gauge where I am or how much more I need to get down in the day. When I use smaller bottles and fill up multiple times I tend to forget. Some of us like smaller portions and refilling. Do what works for you. Thirst cues can sometimes be misinterpreted as hunger cues, so the next time you think you might be hungry, try hydrating *before* snacking. And remember: drinking alcohol and caffeinated beverages can lead to dehydration, so increase your water intake when you indulge.

Pro trick: I use two water bottles. One is for when I will be at home all day. That one is normally a gallon or a half-gallon so when I am done I know I've hit my hydration goal. The second is a thirty-two or forty-ounce to run around with.

Travel hack: I bring my own water bottle from home when I travel so I stay on track. Then I either buy several liters of water at the airport to take to the hotel or I stop at a convenience store on the way to stock up. Hotels seldom have enough water in the room, so we stop to buy a few gallons on the way to our destination. When I am out and about, I carry a sling to hold my water, especially if I am bringing out a bigger bottle.

Ways to make water more appealing: Adding fresh or frozen fruit or even sliced cucumber makes drinking water more colorful and indulgent feeling. Also adding ice in your favorite consistency can be a nice switch-up. Add crushed ice for super cold water. So many people tell me that they have a hard time drinking water, but I promise you, if you begin to consistently do it, you will crave it and almost panic if you don't have your water bottle near.

Balance

I want you to know that I think about food most of the time. I think about how I am going to fuel my body after a workout. I think about if I need to buckle down to get ready for a special occasion. I think about if I want to totally indulge at a dinner party. It's all a choice. And I own it. But in the end I always strive for balance.

For me, nutrition is all about balance. I'll drink a cocktail or two a week but drink plenty of water and green juice. I'll eat good chocolate at night and balance that with hot lemon water in the morning. I move daily and rest daily, embracing all sides of who I am.

While the meat, rice, and gravy meals I grew up on aren't what I eat or feed my family on a regular basis, I can guarantee you that when I visit home I eat it all and still scrape the last bits of gravy off my plate. I believe food is one of the joys of living. If you want the ice cream or bag of chips, be very clear that you are making that choice with no guilt. Enjoy it fully and then get back at it; tomorrow is a new day.

> The secret of your future is hidden in your daily routine.
>
> *Mike Murdock*

——————— RESHAPE WRAP-UP ———————

What you put into your body matters. Food, water, even skincare matters—because what you put on your skin is absorbed into your body.

Listen to your body. What is it telling you? How do you feel after you eat certain foods? Take note of what you eat over a two-week time period, and record how you feel after each meal. This will give you a report telling you if your food choices are serving your body.

I have learned to study food, what is good for me, and how it will enhance my body on a cellular level. When I am eating, I actually think about how I am repairing or healing my body. This mindset makes it easier when a decision time comes for how I make my food choices. It has become fun for me when I know the nutritional properties of a certain vegetable, herb, or protein. It's empowering to know I actually have some control and am participating in the vitality of my health. This is never truer than when I am looking for snack swaps. Swapping my lifelong sweet treats for a healthier version that hits the spot has become a fun pastime.

Living your life and enjoying food must be part of your overall lifestyle. We all know the struggles that surround food for many women. I have worked my whole life to figure out a strategy that works for me when it comes to food—for health reasons and because my job is in front of the camera. I am not willing to deprive myself, but I also know we cannot indulge every day. I have learned a balance for my body type, metabolism, and activity level. This is certainly an area where you cannot compare yourself with anyone else. This is totally a self-discovery practice to find an eating strategy you can live with and feel empowered by.

RESHAPE MOVES ———————————

1. Developing routines around what I put into my body has radically upgraded my overall wellness, but they've also reshaped my mind. When I release the burden of trying to make choices every day and figure out what eating plan I'm on or what supplement I'm taking, it alleviates the daily pressure I used to live under.

2. Preparation is the primary factor in success. If I can't make my green juice in the morning for whatever reason, I keep a few prepackaged clean juices on hand so I don't break my routine. I love to meal prep, and I try to do most of it Sunday night or at the start of the week. At the very least, I'll boil a dozen eggs or make several servings of my chia pudding. We all know that preparation is everything. But it's up to you to figure out your schedule and set yourself up for success.

3. Working with a professional like Sarah Wragge took all the guesswork away for me. Based on my lifestyle, my digestion issues, and my health goals, she gave me the tools necessary to be successful. Educate yourself—find the resources and tools that work for your life. Once you reshape your patterns around food and how you use it, the bliss you'll feel with every bite of a chocolate sundae or each sip of your morning green juice will be a completely new and elevated experience for your mind, heart, soul, and health.

CHAPTER 4

RESHAPE YOUR HEART

A Public Breakup that Led

to a Change of Heart

*Every catastrophe can hand us exactly what
we need to awaken into who we really are.*

ELIZABETH LESSER

Family means everything to me. My parents loved us well, always encouraging me to do my best and giving me the mindset that I could do absolutely anything I dreamed of. They love each other, are dedicated to each other, and are so considerate of each other's needs. I always admired their relationship. I dreamed of a marriage like theirs and a family of my own. I trusted God would make that dream come true in his time—and he did.

Just not in the way I'd imagined.

Prince Charming?

Matters of the heart, the ones that are particularly intimate, have a way of shaping our lives in the most profound ways. I'm sure you've had your own times when your heart felt so much love it could burst and other times when your heart was so broken you would need a whole roll of tape to put it back together.

Have you experienced a time in your life when things were moving so fast you didn't see what was right there in front of you? At a particular point during the early days of my career in Los Angeles, I was working constantly, crisscrossing the country on a weekly basis. I knew it was my time, and I was working hard to build my career and establish myself in the entertainment business on my own merit.

There is much to take in as we grow up during our twenties. We learn how to move through life while we get to know ourselves.

Self-discovery while in the public eye at twenty-five years old added another layer to what we all go through at this time of life, especially when it comes to relationships and matters of the heart.

My cohost for the Miss Teen USA pageant in 1998 was charming, handsome, and Catholic. He was also the most forward guy I'd ever known. He even leaned in to kiss me the first night we met. For me a kiss was a big deal. He was very cool and relaxed about it. I was intrigued but also leery.

When I returned home from the job, a beautiful bouquet of flowers awaited me, sent by my cohost. He was definitely charming. And persuasive.

We began dating. I was still so new to LA, whereas he had lived there for years. He had many friends and knew all the great places to go and see but still liked to hang at home watching movies and made frequent trips to San Diego on weekends to see his family.

When things started to get more serious, I remember asking my girlfriends, "How do you know when someone is 'the one'?"

They said, "You just know."

What worried me was that I didn't "know." He cared deeply for his family, he made me laugh, he said all the right things, he was a hard worker, he was fun. So I chose to focus on those things, even though I heard whisperings of things from other people and I felt deep down he wasn't always being totally honest.

He asked me to marry him after we'd dated a number of years. I always wanted a family and a partnership like my parents had, so I said yes.

I began to plan a wedding and life with my fiancé. I flew to New York to meet with Vera Wang, who designed my wedding gown. We appeared as a couple on *The Oprah Winfrey Show* for an episode about love. The Oprah team wanted to film the wedding to show at a later date. *People* magazine would be covering it. Looking back,

I realize the wedding almost took on a life of its own, getting away from what was really important in a relationship.

Just a week before the wedding, someone close to me shared her concerns about our relationship based on some recent information. My fiancé assured me that what I was told was not true. And I chose to believe him.

I really should have put the brakes on it at that point. I didn't. I wasn't strong enough yet. I was too much of a people pleaser at the time. I thought, *How can I disappoint everyone? My family is flying in to Mexico for this wedding. They have taken off work, spent money on tickets, and everything is in motion.* Even though I knew in my gut that something wasn't right, I pulled myself together and moved forward with the wedding.

Days after the ceremony I was confronted with clear evidence of what I was told prior to the wedding. I felt like the rug had been completely pulled out from under me. In an instant, with no explanation and no apology, everything I thought was true about the last several years of our life together was gone. I can only compare it to a sudden death.

I was heartbroken and confused—betrayed. I knew I had to try to annul the marriage.

Looking back, I could see the red flags so clearly. But I had been so naive. I had a crazy busy career. We ran in different circles. We didn't live together, so I didn't know his comings and goings. I was away in New York once a month and traveled for work. He traveled a lot too. When you work in the entertainment business, that's sometimes how it is.

I remember speaking to one of his friends, trying to understand why. We as women always seem to want to know the *why*. I was with this person for six years, I said, and I wanted to understand. His friend recommended that I move on without an apology or explanation from my ex, because I would never get it or the answers I so desired. That hit me like a ton of bricks. I had to move forward without the expectation of receiving anything from him.

Blinders Off

Most of us have experienced betrayal of some sort. The longer I live, the more I realize that is just a fact. As true as that might be, I'd never wish the experience on anyone. It was as if I'd been in the dark for so long and now I was choosing to take blinders off. The light shone right in my face, nearly blinding me.

It's healthy to feel all your feelings. Trust me, I know that's easier said than done. Medicating them or sweeping them under the rug can become toxic, and I promise you that what you have not dealt with will show up in some way down the road. So be uncomfortable, sit in the pain, and *feel*.

I felt all my feelings. I cried a lot. I'd cry myself to sleep, waking up with a headache and eyes practically swollen shut. I'd remember things that had happened and try to figure out where I'd gone wrong, waking up in the middle of the night thinking everything was normal and then being faced with the cruel reality of this betrayal.

Thank God for my sister Gena, who was right there with me, my rock. She didn't leave my side for months. She was supportive, compassionate, and strong. We'd talk and talk and talk. She listened more than anything, but she's wise. She always gave me such great advice. It was the therapy I needed, having someone who loved me unconditionally and was totally there for me. I will be forever grateful to her for showing up for me the way she did during that time. I couldn't have gotten through it without her.

Talking about it with my sister and my friends was, in a way, like vomiting up all the bad stuff. When I was finally empty, a kind of grace settled in. I wanted better for myself. I'd been in this relationship for years. How had I been so blind? I needed to figure out how I'd gotten to this place. Though it was clear he'd been deceptive, I needed to figure out what part I'd played in this. I was going to identify the mentality and self-talk in myself that had contributed to this outcome, that had negatively influenced my future and the possibility of the husband and marriage I asked God for.

I not only felt all my feelings, but I gave them names. When I recognized a feeling as "feeling betrayed," the question became, *If not betrayal, what do I want to feel?* I'd listen for the answer coming from deep, deep inside my heart: *I want to feel valued and cherished.*

Then: *If that's what you want, Ali, where are you going to get that feeling? Could it ever come from the relationship you were in?* It became clear to me that I'd been spared a lifetime of disappointment. While the heartbreak was hard, it was also a blessing. I began to change, and I flipped the switch on my thoughts.

I didn't want to become a bitter, angry, resentful person. I wanted to move on in a way that was positive and healthy. I needed to figure out how to heal.

My heart was getting a reshape.

Tethered

When life turns upside down, you can feel dizzy and off-balance, like you're falling. What I found is that it helps to tether yourself to what you know to be true in your core. For me, that's my faith.

I began to pray like never before. Only God could comfort me and give me the peace and healing I so desired and transform my heart. God was present for me. It has been the only time in my life that I

> To trust God in the light is nothing, but to trust him in the dark—that is faith.
>
> *Charles H. Spurgeon*

heard God's voice so clearly, and I think it is because I was so fully dependent on him. My friend Davia gave me a student Bible—a terrific gift because it really comforted me and helped me to dig in and learn. I read from it every day. When an emotion would come up—like anger, for instance, which bubbled up a lot during this time—I would search for passages that spoke about it. After reading, I was immediately covered in peace, knowing that all I needed to do was to continue to seek God and he would take care of the rest.

Surrendered Heart

I begged God to walk alongside me and help me put one foot in front of the other, to help me move forward in my life in the best possible way. I prayed: *Help me, because I don't trust myself. I made such a horrible mistake, trying to do this my way. Show me your way, God. From here on out, I give my life to you, in faith, because I know that through you all things are possible and your plan for my life is so much better than anything I could dream up on my own.*

I spent so many months trying to make sense of it all. I barely ate anything. I couldn't turn on the TV because all I could hear were lies and untruths wrapped in shiny things coming back at me through the screen. So I surrendered. I had no idea what was next for me. I just trusted and prayed for months, all in. During that time, I did a lot of reflection and centering. I now like to refer to it as heart work.

I asked myself many hard questions: *Who am I, and what kind of life do I want? What are my heart's true desires?* It became clear to me that I had a new opportunity to get it right this time, and I was not going to mess that up. So I journaled, pouring my feelings out on the page, being very specific about what I wanted in a future partner, asking the hard questions and listening, searching God for answers and asking him to bring that person to me—the man he wanted for me.

The Best Thing

I know with everything in my being that God gave me many signs along the way to get out of the relationship, but I wouldn't listen. In the end, he had to force a reshape on me. It was divine, Fatherly. He was saying "No! This is not the plan I have for your life," and his large hand swooped in and grabbed me out of that relationship. I didn't have the ability to see that I was settling, so God closed that door for me.

It was painful, but I understand now that so much growth happens through pain if you allow it to teach you. Good experiences, while delightful, don't lead to growth in themselves. Pain was revealing who I truly was. I see pain differently than I did before. I don't love pain but absolutely do want to be transformed, *reshaped*.

That's the heart of it, right there. Heartbreak forced me to go on an interior journey to transformation. And that was a gift!

Blame Game

The hardest part of it all was trying to pick up the pieces and heal while the other person seemed to have moved on without a second thought.

For me to move toward being whole again, I knew I needed to forgive. But if I forgave him, wouldn't I be saying that what he did was okay? My whole being told me that it wasn't okay. So I spoke to priests, theologians, therapists, friends, and mentors to help me wrap my head around what forgiveness meant in my situation.

What I came away with from those conversations is that forgiveness isn't a blank check. It's a way of releasing those negative feelings of pain, resentment, and anger and trusting that what happens is not my responsibility. I have to trust God with the outcome.

Okay, that sounds great on paper, but try to make your heart feel that! While my mind understood the concept, it still was not settling into my heart. Then I heard this: Holding on to hurt, pain, resentment, and anger harms the wounded, not the offender. Forgiveness frees us to live in the present. Reliving the wrong that was done to us keeps us living in the past and missing today's beauty.

Now, this actually landed on me! It spoke to every fiber of my being. I wanted to live fully in the present, notice God's beauty all around me, and not take any of that negative baggage into the relationship I was confident that God was going to deliver to me. God began reshaping my heart when I surrendered to forgiveness. This heart reshape allowed me to process what happened to me, let go of bitterness, and live in the present moment.

So, I forgave—without an apology. And to this day I hold no resentment toward him. I am actually grateful, and if I ever ran into him, I would say thank you. I wish him well but hope he doesn't do what he did to me to anyone else.

A lesson I have learned is that when someone betrays you, hurts you, says untruths about you, it is a reflection of *their* character, not yours. And when any type of betrayal shows up, yes, I am initially hurt, but I soon remember this and am able to give that person a little grace, knowing that it is coming from some sort of angst within them. I am actually able to have compassion for that person.

Turning Point

Though life wasn't turning out the way I'd imagined it would or wanted it to, by making myself present and open, I received tremendous grace. God hadn't given me my dream of marriage and family yet, but in his time, I would love again with my whole heart.

The hard days got a little easier. Slowly, rays of sunshine started to come through. I made a conscious choice to do the work necessary to become whole and be open to who God had in my future. The stillness and the pain ended up being my greatest teachers. I dug into my faith, reading and journaling, discovering deeper parts of myself. *The Purpose Driven Life Journal* was my companion. Each day I would read a passage and write down what I felt as I read, trying to relate it to my own situation. It was healing work.

I remember writing daily at the top of each page in my journal exactly what I wanted in a future relationship. I wrote that I wanted to find a man whom I respected and who would hold my heart gently and always care for it. Also I wrote to protect myself—so if something or someone came into my life that wasn't that, it would be very clear. What had seemed like the worst time in my life began to feel like the absolute best. I was choosing to walk though my life in full awareness, blinders off, with no illusions, for the first time. Sure, I felt wobbly at first. I didn't really trust myself in the beginning, but I asked God to hold my hand and guide me. I'd made so many mistakes in the past, and I didn't want to do it alone anymore. I love the old saying, "If you want to make God laugh, tell him your plans."

I'd had a good start, a loving family, and a healthy childhood before becoming a public figure. Coming from a small town, I'd felt my whole town was depending on me, looking to me to be the representative of Louisiana to the world. That was intense. I was determined to live up to that responsibility.

My quick marriage and annulment led to a huge change in me. It was a birth, in a way. Viewed from where I am now, I see it almost as my beginning. The intensely public breakup was the first trauma I'd ever endured. It was an opportunity, I thought, to truly grow. It opened up my interior world. I began to really understand grace.

True Heart's Desire

My time with God during this period stoked in me a desire to learn more. I signed up for a theology class as a way to go deeper into my faith. That's where I met Alejandro.

My friend Eduardo Verástegui and I were auditioning for a film together. He told me about a class being taught by theologian and lawyer, Leo Severino. The name of it was Going Deeper. I thought, *That's exactly what I need!* Once I got to know Leo, he asked me to come speak at a youth retreat. I immediately agreed. Leo offered to get me a ride with his friend, Alejandro Monteverde, so I wouldn't have to make the long drive alone.

I saw what a man of honor and character Alejandro was right away. In my journals I'd poured out my hopes to meet a man of such character. He had humility, passion for his work and his family, and a deep spiritual life. I admired him and I respected him. I'd prayed fervently for months about what I had versus what I wanted, and now here he was, the embodiment of the qualities I'd prayed for. I often say that God delivered Alejandro right to me, and he opened up my heart to a whole new love, something I never thought possible for myself.

I enjoyed talking with someone with such an intense creative and spiritual life. Our romance truly bloomed out of mutual respect. We were intentional about waiting to be intimate until we were married. I needed to get to know him completely before committing in any way. We closed down a lot of restaurants in LA, talking late into the night. That was the best thing we could have ever done for our relationship. There was no sense in which we were fooling or charming each other. We both knew each other's hearts and minds before we knew each other intimately. When we consummated our relationship on our wedding night, we both knew we were bonded for life.

My husband and I are not perfect humans; no one is. But what I do know is that he was an answer to my prayers, delivered to me. He's trustworthy and kind. But what's more important is that he leads our family and is our biggest protector and supporter. He makes sure we're in church every single Sunday and he reminds us to bring gratitude into every day, to always put God first, being fully faithful and surrendering to his plan. He has high standards for himself, and he's always trying to be better, do better. When you have someone like that in your life, it makes you want to be better too. He's the most incredible partner for me. I don't think I would be in the place where I am without him. I feel like he is my gift from God.

When I think back on those early days, I try to have compassion on the younger version of me and the choices I made that led to heartbreak. I no longer make space in my life for people who are not dedicated to honesty and growth. Even though I consider myself a people person, my circle has gotten smaller as I've gotten older, and I think that's a good thing. I would never want to go back to my twenties or thirties. I know myself, and I like myself. I don't worry as much, and I've learned to surrender to life's lessons.

I thank God every day that he brought Alejandro and me together.

How amazing to think that it all started from something so horrible and difficult. Isn't that kind of beautiful?

Sharing from the Heart

Every heart is constantly being shaped. The question is, what shape is yours headed toward? Is it growing to allow room for the right people and for more love? Or is it hardening and shrinking? Or has it stopped growing and changing altogether?

We, as women, don't talk about our emotional state that often. We tend to push through because we have so many areas of responsibility. But we have all had moments in our lives that can abruptly shift us, those moments when life changes forever. Through both triumph and difficulty, we can let the experiences grow us into the very best versions of ourselves. But that decision comes from the heart—especially when the difficult moments turn our worlds upside down. When we hold on to hurt, pain, resentment, and anger, it harms us far more than it harms the offender. Forgiveness frees us to live in the present. Reliving the wrong that was done to us keeps us living in the past and missing today's beauty. We've all been through some type of heartbreak in our lives. The question is, how long are we going to sit in that? And how are we going to choose to move through it? I think we need to feel the feelings and process what happened, but there will come a time—a time only you know—when you need to get up and begin the mending process. I knew I did not want to close up and harden my heart.

Our emotional state can become unbalanced by emotional stress, unforgiveness, a hurt from tragedy or loss, a heartbreak, or unresolved childhood experiences. Whatever your situation may be that is keeping your heart from flowing the way it should, I can tell you that if you really do the work, it will change the course of your life.

There is a verse that says, "Guard your heart, for everything you do flows from it" (Proverbs 4:23). This is wisdom to live by, and it has become a baseline for what I let into my heart and what I keep out.

Reshapes for the heart take effort and dedication, but all good things in life do. Start with the basics, journaling your feelings. There is no order to journaling; just write and get it all out of your heart and out of your head. You may want to start with listing the desires of your heart. This is the first step to release. It can be very difficult to go there and pull it out of yourself, but it's necessary. Getting your feelings out is always step one. For me looking for qualified spiritual guidance was life changing; it allowed me to place my emotions with God. This was a big turning point for me. I no longer had to carry any of it around with me; it was released, and I trusted God at his word.

I'll never forget having a massage during the mending time of my heart, and for the entire time of the massage, I wept. It felt so good to release all I had been carrying. On another day I went to a workout class with a friend, and at the end, the instructor had us lie on the floor and put our hands over our hearts to thank our bodies for the workout. In that moment I felt in touch with myself and experienced another release, and I just broke down and started crying. You've got to get it out and let it go!

You must position yourself to let it go. Perhaps it's traditional therapy, finding a support group, opening up to your significant other or closest friend, doing the things in life that bring joy to your heart, stepping away from those who have caused your heart to ache, or finding your peaceful place in nature where you can release it all.

For me, using *The Five Minute Journal* is a meaningful daily activity that has impacted the overall quality of my life. I use it as a place to speak out about what I am grateful for; in essence it has become my gratitude journal. Thinking of things you are grateful for, writing them down and speaking them out, actually rewires your brain. These daily practices are not just therapy mumbo jumbo; they actually work!

Once you heal those hurts and reshape your heart, you no longer need to look outside yourself for fulfillment or self-medicate. You stop thinking about the "things" that will make you momentarily happy and you instead become settled with yourself. We often hear about various techniques and professional strategies for dealing with matters of the heart. Whichever way connects with you, use it; just get started and don't look back!

—————— RESHAPE WRAP-UP ——————

Don't let the pain, disappointment, or missteps from your past steal your future. Value yourself enough to listen to your heart; sit in your situation to feel your feelings; commit to the process; and set yourself up to let it go. You are worth every tear you shed and every feeling you need to feel to move through and beyond the bondage of what has kept you locked up.

Trusting God with every part of your heart takes time, but I guarantee it will reshape your heart in a way that clears out all the hurt, pain, disappointment, and heartache that has been keeping you from living to your full potential. It is life changing at the deepest levels.

We are all guilty of self-medicating in some way for different reasons; we've used food, shopping, substances, entertainment, and relationships to avoid ourselves. Stand up for yourself and identify what you are doing and why. Seek the support and resources you need to begin your reshape. This is not easy work, and you can't do it halfway. You need to commit to yourself that you are all in. Once you start to feel the emotional release, a peace washes over you, and there is no turning back. You are on your way.

RESHAPE MOVES ──────────────────

1. Write down your feelings and journal daily, either in a notebook or in the notes on your phone. You may be surprised at the way this task naturally pulls out your deepest thoughts. Be honest, but also positive, taking ownership of your thoughts, decisions, and actions. *The Purpose Driven Life Journal* gave me a biblical prompt that I was able to draw from and journal about my own situation.

2. Pain can be a door to a life transformation, and often forgiveness is the key that opens the door for your reshape. Take the time to study and understand the concept of forgiveness and how it becomes your own personal superpower.

3. I repeat this prayer, drawing on the words of Martin Luther King Jr., in my daily meditation: "Use me, God. Show me how to take who I am, who I want to be, and what I can do, and use it for a purpose greater than myself." Perhaps this prayer or one created from your heart will help bring order to your mind and open your heart in a new way.

CHAPTER 5

RESHAPE YOUR ENVIRONMENT

Curating Spaces to Live

Your Best Life

I'm going to make everything around me beautiful—that will be my life.

ELSIE DE WOLFE

I'm super social, but I'm also a homebody—home means the world to me. So staying put in the house I'd bought with my ex was not an option. Part of moving *on* would mean moving *out*. My heart was healing, but I realized that to fully heal I needed to create a home of my own. I started to look for a new place to live. Without my even asking, my mom came from Louisiana to help.

Growing up, I loved watching my mom work in her beauty salon. It was always so entertaining. Customers, who were basically like family, would come in and download everything that was going on with their families. Then the transformations would begin. I always noticed a hopeful look in their eyes—an excited anticipation. You probably know what I mean. To this day I still get that feeling when I sit in a salon chair! Customers walked out looking terrific, but it wasn't just their hair that had changed. Their whole countenance was brighter. I loved watching that transformation. I'm sure I spent a thousand hours in that beauty salon just watching my mom do hair.

There was lots of mischief in that salon too—so many fun times, with me trying to cut and color my friends' hair or vice versa. My job was to clean the shop, which I did not like. I'd get one of my friends or siblings to help. We'd sweep up, then splash a bucketful of hot water and soap on the floor and put washrags on our feet as we pretended we were Olympic skaters. Or we would get on our hands and knees and push off one wall, sliding across the floor to the other wall. Little pieces of hair covered us from head to toe. I am not sure how clean I ever got that shop, but I definitely turned a boring chore into something so fun. I guess I was "reshaping" even then.

While Dad was working on his week out in the oil fields, we took the opportunity to go out and visit friends, run errands, or just get out of the house. Mom always had a project—usually helping someone. She's the most industrious woman you could ever meet. If a friend wanted to wallpaper her bathroom, Mom would be right there hanging wallpaper, and you could bet it was done right. If you wanted to lay a wood floor, refurbish an antique piece of furniture, or just find new throw pillows for your couch, my mom was the one you called. She always showed up for people, and I've admired her so much for that.

Her creativity was boundless. I'd see something cool in a magazine that I wanted to try, and she'd say, "We can do that." She'd figure out a way. I honestly do not remember ever buying a dress at a store. Christmas dresses, prom dresses—they were always made by a local seamstress, and they were amazing. Inspiration was found sometimes in magazines, sometimes on television, or sometimes we would head to the fabric store to page through book after book of the latest patterns. Once we landed on a design, we'd pick out the fabric and all the trim. I learned so much through that process, finding the perfect colors and textures that complemented one another. My mom was creative, and this was one of the outlets that gave her such joy. I loved seeing the satisfaction on her face when we went out with those dresses and received compliments. That taught me that in life you should do things that feed your soul and nourish that little part inside of you that sometimes gets forgotten because life happens.

When it came to costumes, Mom went all out. Once, she made me the most amazing turtle costume. She built the shell out of chicken wire and papier-mâché. She dressed me in a green unitard with a green swim cap and painted my face, then rolled me into the competition on a dolly. We won! Any project, anything for school, I always won first place because of my mom. I definitely got my creative and competitive spirit from her.

Building a Life

Because of Mom, I grew up appreciating beautiful environments, especially homes. My mom didn't have an abundance of money to spend on her surroundings, but she didn't let that stand in her way. She was a DIY queen before that was even a thing! She didn't mind getting down to the studs to get things the way she wanted them. She could do everything from painting to spackling to paneling to wallpapering. I have never seen her with a project she couldn't tackle. If an area in our home no longer served her needs, she'd tackle it with abandon and make it useful and beautiful. She not only did this for herself, but she did it for all her friends, and always on a budget. To help realize their dreams, she'd roll up her sleeves and get to work. I grew up witnessing that.

My mom curated every detail of her home, and I was taking note. She lovingly created a home our family felt proud of, and she shared it with friends and family. I learned that from her. When I walk into a room, I notice every single detail, and not just visually. I experience spaces on an emotional level. The lighting, the smells, the sounds, the textures—I experience all of it, taking it all in. My senses are on alert. I'll notice the detailing in the millwork, the upholstery, the window treatments, the pottery sitting on a shelf—everything. Friends who've redone a room or bought a new house or renovated love to invite me over because I notice every single little thing. I think I am so passionate about it because our home is part of our personal story, where past, present, and future come together.

When I was in high school, most of the girls took home economics classes, where they learned to cook and keep house. I took industrial arts instead. I had a goal of building my own furniture. And I did! My high school bedroom was furnished with custom-made furniture: my bed, a chair, and a dresser were all Ali Landry originals. The fact that I was fifteen and handling a table saw is something I'm still pretty proud of. I had the coolest room a teenager could want. When I grew up and moved out of that room, my mom helped me create my next living space. She and my dad have been there for every single move since. To this day we are in sync. We talk about how pieces should be refinished, figure out color palettes, and consider what accessories best complement the space. Today, as I look around my home, I sense her with me in big and little ways. Her passion for reshaping a home has become my own.

The Mood of a Place

When I am creating, I am happy. I sense that little voice inside that says, *That's it—do more of that.* My drive to create and cultivate beautiful spaces grew out of my relationship with my mother. It's a lifelong pursuit and passion for me. I'm always trying to hone my knowledge and my instincts. I can remember wanting to be an archaeologist when I was younger, and I think that was because of my love of lost things and knowing and understanding their stories. I loved to visit antique stores; I dreamed of buying some of the pieces because I felt like their story was still inside of them, and I wanted that story to continue in my life. I'd save my money to buy *Architectural Digest* and swoon over all of the beautiful interiors and architecture around the world. I would tear out all of my favorite images and save them in a big bin for years.

When I bought my first home, I referred to all of those pages, drawing inspiration and really trying to understand why I was moved by them. Was the emotion it evoked from looking at it as a whole, or was it the individual pieces that drew me in? Creating inviting spaces is self-expression for me, just like it is for my mom. I also really appreciate the beauty of imperfection and using humble things in a space, like branches, stones, or driftwood the kids find on the beach. Bringing nature in makes the space feel grounded.

While I'm very deliberate about my environment, I believe all of us are constantly taking cues from our environments. We have varying degrees of awareness of what makes us feel comfortable and inspired or uncomfortable and uninspired. Imagine walking into a room where the lighting is poor—maybe it's fluorescent—or it smells musty and damp. It's hard to ignore the brain signals telling you something is unpleasant.

Beautiful surroundings are relaxing. The brain subconsciously notices that all is well and says, *All right, then, it's safe to settle in and relax.*

Unique to Me

A comfortable, beautiful home invites me and everyone who enters to relax and be present. I also want it to feel unique and special, transporting. I want things around me that, as Marie Kondo says, "spark joy."

I'm most attracted to pieces crafted with intention and care. They don't have to be "perfect"—in fact, pieces with a story and a history are rarely flawless. I love special things that have been passed down in our family. It's also really special when I can look around and see hints of where I've been—little mementos. When I'm on an adventure I keep that in mind. If I see something that delights me,

I think, *Would this serve well in our home and also remind me of this special trip?*

Editing a Space

That said, if I'm surrounded by visual clutter, my thoughts feel cluttered. At one point when the kids were younger I remember our house feeling so full. We had collected so much stuff having three little ones that every drawer was a mess, every closet packed. Our home was bursting at the seams, and I felt like that mess spilled over into my life. I couldn't think straight. It was affecting my mental state. My brain felt like a jumbled mess, and I couldn't focus or complete any one task fully. It was past time to reshape our space.

> Maybe the life you've always wanted is buried under everything you own!
>
> *Joshua Becker*

I began to frequently purge things that were no longer useful, giving them away to charity or handing them over to somebody who could use them. This is especially true of kids' things! It turns out that less really is more.

I began to release what didn't bring joy.

Now I try to hold things lightly rather than grasp them tightly.

When embarking on an environment reshape, try putting a pause on impulsive purchases. Commit to investing in pieces you love, especially things you use and see every day. Sure, it may take a little more effort to find and it may cost more, but you're worth it! By buying fewer things that are of higher quality, you'll be surrounding yourself with the message, "You are worth it!"

Over time, you'll find you're accumulating less. Ask yourself if you need it. Why do you want it? Will buying it bring fleeting pleasure that will quickly fade, or will it bring you happiness and joy for years to come?

For example, I choose to buy goat's-milk soap infused with essential oils from the farmers' market rather than supermarket soap. Though it is a bit more time consuming to go to the farmers' market for soap, the simple act of washing my hands—essentially a mundane thing—becomes an occasion that sparks joy for me, and I know that the goat's milk is good for me down to the cellular level. Mindfully choosing what's in your environment can make a big difference in your daily routines!

Inviting Moments

Another motivator for me is creating opportunities for peaceful moments. We rarely sat still when our children were younger. Now that they are a little older, my husband and I can sit and talk and enjoy life. It's lovely to have places to relax and sit comfortably, either alone or for a chat. There's something so inviting about a side table and chair where a candle waits alongside a book of matches, begging to be lit. The morning light glistening across the kitchen table as you have your first cup of coffee. I work at my desk and can look out a window at the leaves dancing on the olive trees, it's the little nook that promises a peaceful moment of reading while bossa nova spills out of the speakers. When you have those kinds of spaces around the house, it's a hopeful feeling—an invitation to linger and enjoy.

It's the simple things that bring me joy, the things that don't cost a dime that feed my spirit.

What Do You Treasure?

Not long ago my husband and I packed up our kids early one morning for a day at "the happiest place on earth": Disneyland. We spent a beautiful day together making memories. When we arrived back home after dark, we were shocked. The new house we'd only been in for a few months had been burglarized. Thank God no one had been in the house and no one was hurt. Even so, it was truly upsetting.

Someone had broken in through the balcony off our master bedroom. In that room I'd kept special valuables, things I really cared for, in keepsake trays. The thieves completely emptied those trays. All my jewelry and many sentimental pieces were gone. Everything from my finer pieces to my grandmother's costume jewelry from the forties, passed on to me. They'd also taken a Miraculous Medal depicting the Blessed Virgin Mary that was precious to me. They'd taken the piece of my mom's wedding dress that I'd pinned inside of my own on my wedding day. Even my kids' umbilical cords were gone. It was so sad!

But after the shock and sadness wore off, I realized these things, these beautiful things that meant so much, were simply physical items. They're not what matters most to me. What matters most aren't objects at all. What I treasure most is my family: my marriage and three beautiful children. I get excited about aesthetics and art and curating a beautiful home, but things don't bring true joy. What brings me joy is my family, my relationship with God, and connecting with women to inspire lasting change. Those connections happen in person or even here in this book. I love how lives are being touched as we share to make our lives richer. That's what I truly value. Ultimately it is a connection—making myself vulnerable and sharing the struggles and how I've come out on the other side, and trusting that another human who possibly relates to my experience can do the same for themselves. I've learned that we must speak from the heart to touch the heart.

Still Dreaming

I've stretched my creativity a lot over the years, reshaping my environment in big and small ways. I never get tired of trying or learning new things, researching, and figuring out what works for me now.

For the past few years I have been dreaming about a little beach house that we just finished building in Mexico. A home by the ocean has always been one of my husband's greatest dreams. Buying this property was such a leap of faith, and the only reason we did it was because circumstances showed us that life is short, every moment is precious, and tomorrow is not promised. This project is so important to us because it is a complete reflection of our souls. It represents the way we want to live—intentional, thoughtful, connected to nature and the world around us. It's a place where we have the blessing to look out at the expanse of the ocean, where the sky touches the strength, the fluidity, and the depth of the sea. It's so vast, instilling in my heart that there is something much bigger than I am. It forces me to get outside of myself and my mind and feel that connection to something greater, to *God*. It warms my heart—thinking about the joy we'll experience there as a family and with friends.

I have invested hours and hours and hours—years, really—researching. I dug into the work of architects and designers and searched for meaningful historical pieces and antiques. It's been a joy going deep into this process. I've visualized every single corner.

I have so many Pinterest boards for every single room in this house! Dreaming and planning for it makes me feel energized. It represents the next step of my journey of reshaping my physical environment. I've never been more purposeful than I have been on this project.

While I am not an interior designer or architect by trade, I love it so much and I get a sense of fulfillment when I tap into that side of myself. Never give up on your passions or what gives you joy! Those passions are there for a reason.

Now, how about you? Could your environment use a reshape?

Changing up your physical environment can invigorate you. It'll give you a fresh perspective.

Is your house a home? Are you happy being there and living in it? Is it a space that truly represents you? Are you proud of it? Is it set up to provide structure and motivation for your life? It's not about the amount of money you have to spend on things or a remodel. Work with what you have and be thoughtful about it. Oprah tells the story that when she was only making $22,000 per year, she would save a few dollars every week for fresh flowers in her home because of how it made her feel; it gave her true joy. These little things around the home create contentment in the soul and a sense of peace in the spirit. Creating your personal environment will give you life rather than steal it. That is the ultimate reshape.

How do you feel in your space? What do you see when you look around? Are you inspired to live your best life in there? Maybe one area needs a reshape, or maybe your entire home needs a total refresh. The goal is to work as you can to make progress. The edit always comes first for me—removing the things no longer needed. Donate or sell these on Facebook Marketplace. Look at your space and see if you can simply reposition furniture or repurpose a room that is no longer serving your or your family's needs. Sometime a fresh coat of paint, or fixing things around the house that need maintenance and you have been putting off, can breathe new life into your space. Perhaps you'll put some organizational systems in place or declutter your closest, clean out a pantry, re-cover furniture, buy a lounge chair and umbrella for your patio, or choose a new rug and pillows—those basics can very much reshape your day-to-day, clearing your mind and settling your heart. Nothing is worse than dealing with the pressures of the world and coming home to a space that doesn't give you what you need it to.

What is your vibe? What textures, colors, scents, and overall look make you light up inside? I love to look through design magazines, watch home makeover shows, scroll through Pinterest, and dream about the most perfect space custom designed just for me. I love to bring the outside in—for instance, with a couple of special crystals and rocks we have collected. I bring in outside plant clippings to make arrangements for my home, and I have planted an herb garden that we can use year-round in California. We have defined places in our home where all five of us can gather together. Just as important is space for when we need private time. I keep a list of chores for myself and the kids so we can keep our space tidy. If we go for a few days with no upkeep, cleaning becomes a major task; I'm sure you've been there. I'd rather not have that looming over my head.

Our personal environment often gets overlooked with the hustle of life. Yet this is the place our life flows through. We owe it to ourselves to design spaces purposefully with our particular lifestyles in mind.

So get out the paintbrush, hang some new artwork, get a garbage bag or two and fill them, have a yard sale, or just organize your shoes and purses and move along. This reshape will boost your life in every area: heart, mind, soul, and health.

—— RESHAPE WRAP-UP ——

Listen to that little voice inside yourself that rejoices when you are doing something you love. Do more of that.

Your space is either helping you feel joy and contentment or it's a source of discomfort and strain on your life. Design spaces that are not only functional and give you order but are representative of you. Your space should be meaningful to your heart, mind, soul, and health.

Reshaping by editing and clearing out the clutter is a must. Clutter around you physically creates clutter in your mind. No one has time for that.

RESHAPE MOVES ——————

1. Go room by room in your space. Make a list of what's working and what's not. Create a plan and a schedule for how you are going to approach this reshape. Start with the basics: clear out the clutter. Then move to the design: functionality and aesthetics. Build a budget and start small. Once you see and feel yourself in this reshaped space, it will inspire you to do more.

2. Make a list of the most valued treasures in your home. Are they sitting in the back of a closet, or are they out and displayed for you to appreciate and help keep a memory close? These treasures are what can give you that boost of energy or serenity. Figure out the best way to showcase your mementos. Your things are meant to be enjoyed, not packaged away waiting for a particular time in your life.

3. Again, let Pinterest be your friend. Create a vision board of colors, textures, furniture styles, and room flow.

4. Playlists are great too. I love to create a playlist of music that creates a mood that I'd like in my home. It helps draw me in when I am looking for inspiration.

CHAPTER 6

RESHAPE THROUGH PAIN

How Tragedy Reshaped My Soul

I have made you and I will carry you; I will
sustain you and I will rescue you.

ISAIAH 46:4

One thing's for certain: we all experience pain at some point in our lives.

Pain isn't something any of us want or seek out. But pain comes along even while living a full and beautiful life. I refuse to settle for a stagnant life, so I welcome transformation even though it can be painful—at times even agonizing. I've found my way back to joy with interior work. I say "work" because, honestly, it was not easy. It took patience. I had to sit with the pain and not medicate it. It took persistence. And it took faith.

Transformation can be like walking through fire. It's scary, and sometimes you can't see what's right in front of you. But stepping out of the fire and into fresh air makes your next breath feel sweet and delicious. That's how I see pain. It makes life's smallest joys even more precious.

Learning a New Language

For as long as I can remember, I've enjoyed exploring new places and meeting new people. When I go someplace new, I feel that new place expanding my heart, igniting my creativity, and renewing my energy. Every destination is a chance to grow, to learn, to gain a new perspective and expand my horizons. Each new place is a start of something new.

One of my favorite destinations is San Miguel de Allende. It's a truly magical city in central Mexico. When I visited the city briefly on a road trip with Alejandro and his family when we were dating, I fell in love with the place. I knew I wanted to return.

So when the sitcom television show I'd been working on, called *Eve*, went on hiatus, I decided to seize the day and go back to that beautiful city. Though we weren't officially engaged, Alejandro and I knew we were going to get married. Because his family only spoke Spanish, it was very important to me to learn the language to be able to communicate with them. I only knew *hola*—"hello"—in Spanish. That was it. I learned there was a small Spanish school in San Miguel de Allende where I could study the language. I began to plan my personal *Eat, Pray, Love* journey.

As I was setting everything up, Alejandro said, "I don't think you should go alone." I said, "I'm a grown woman. I'll be fine!" But he said, "I'd like to send my parents with you." I didn't really know his parents that well, and we couldn't even communicate at that point. But he was adamant. His mom loved to travel, and his dad was retired and pretty flexible. He spoke to them and they agreed to be my roommates for a month in San Miguel de Allende. This was incredible to me. How kind of them to just drop everything to come and watch over me while I had my adventure in the charming Spanish colonial town. I flew in from Los Angeles, and they came from the coast to meet me there. Together we settled in for four weeks of domestic adventure together in this magical city of doors.

The Jewel of Latin America

One thing that struck me right away was how walkable the city is. You don't have to drive. People walk everywhere. The fairytale-like cobblestone streets are lined with shops and homes featuring brightly colored, gorgeous doors and red geraniums in pots lining the upper terraces. Their facades are painted in vivid colonial colors—deep burgundy reds, mustard yellows, or dark blue. And it's a deeply spiritual town with more than three hundred churches and reminders of the faith everywhere you look. I could hardly believe such a place existed—it was all so picturesque and vibrant that it seemed perfectly appropriate when it was named the World's Best City in *Travel and Leisure*'s World's Best Awards two years in a row. I fell right into step there and lived just like a local.

Our apartment was in the city's historic center, literally in the shadow of the Parroquia de San Miguel Arcángel, a neo-Gothic cathedral with intricately crafted pink towers. Seeing that church every day was glorious—a glimpse into the artful soul of the city.

Everywhere we went, the most wonderful artists were creating something beautiful, tasty, or precious. Walking along, you might see a painter with an easel set up in the middle of the street painting the centuries-old cathedral a mile in the distance. We met creative people from all over the world there. It's definitely an artist's dream, whether you're a visual artist or a creator of culinary delights. Since it's an international city, you find the most incredible chefs from all over the world. Entrepreneurs looking for a slower-paced life love it as well, like the couple I met from Paris who'd opened a little French café down the street from our apartment where I would visit weekly for the croissants and who later made my wedding cake.

Living with my future in-laws gave us a chance to get to know one another. Alejandro's mom is very social and loves to be with people. She's traveled all over the world—still does, to this day—with her friends and her sons. It's her passion. She's a really strong woman. From the start, something about her reminded me of my grandmother on my dad's side of the family—she even resembled her.

Alejandro's dad was one of the most special people I have ever met. He had the most beautiful heart imaginable—such a loving and affectionate man, but also a jokester. The two of them took care of me. They were so nurturing. I love how I grew up, but my parents raised me to be independent and do my own thing. Alejandro's parents are different. They cooked for me, worried over me, and looked out for me in everything I did.

Rituals of Family Life

The three of us quickly fell into comforting rituals. In the mornings I would walk to school with Alejandro's mom. I was there to learn Spanish, so I chose not to hang out with the American students so much. Instead, I spent time with the locals and my in-laws. My strategy worked too. I learned more quickly by speaking only Spanish. I wouldn't always say the right word, and sometimes I'd use the wrong tense. But Alejandro's parents were gentle with me and really appreciated my efforts to learn their language. Gradually, I started to get it. I knew the language was taking hold in me when I started dreaming in Spanish.

I would finish school about 12:30, and sure enough, Alejandro's dad was always waiting for me promptly by the door after class every day. He'd greet me and away we would go to the market behind the school—booth after booth offering fresh vegetables, cheeses, fresh meat, fruit drinks, and everything we needed for dinner that night. That was our ritual. We'd buy mole for our chicken from one woman, we'd buy cheese from another, whatever was needed. After we'd shopped at the market, we'd go back and cook and eat. Then we'd have a siesta. Everybody there took a siesta! During the hottest part of the day, taking a rest was pure bliss.

After siesta his mom and I would get our exercise by exploring the twenty-four blocks of the city. On one of our walks I got to know all the shop owners and vendors. I even made friends with a Realtor who took us to visit the most incredible homes, restored to perfection and super authentic, furnished by local artisans. The Realtor took us behind those magical doors to see some of the most beautiful, restored properties I had ever seen. In the evenings, we'd go into the town square, which was right in front of Parroquia de San Miguel Arcángel. Everyone gathered there at night. There'd be musicians playing and painters painting, vendors selling *elote* (corn) or creative varieties of *paletas*—the icy, spicy, Mexican delight in every flavor imaginable, even *cerveza* (beer). It was all amazing to me. As we took in the sights, I told her, "I love this place! I'd love to get married here."

The architecture and design of the place sparked something in me. I just fell in love with it. It wasn't long before I knew every single street. Those homes inspired me. I got so many ideas that I later used in my own home. The colors I chose for the paint, the landscaping, the fixtures, the lanterns, the tiles—I can trace all of it back to inspirations I got in San Miguel.

While we walked in the evenings, my future father-in-law sat at the center of the park making friends. I've never met anyone like him. He exuded light and love. If music was playing, he'd dance—I mean really dance, even going into the splits like James Brown. If there was a bicycle, he would get on it and ride it backward. He would do handstands—he'd do anything for an audience. And he was a jokester—always smiling and making others laugh.

He carried a leather briefcase with him wherever he went. Inside were pictures of his children and grandchildren plus newspaper clippings featuring the opening of this son's restaurant or that son's new movie. It was like his mobile scrapbook. He was so proud! So, nine out of ten times, when we circled back to meet him in the park, we'd find him talking with someone, with that briefcase open, sharing pictures and telling stories about his family. Everybody who met him fell in love with him. He was effusive, funny, and full of life. He was fiercely protective and loved with abandon. Even though I didn't always understand everything he said, I knew his heart. You could see it. To this day I recall how his face lit up with that big smile. I came to love the sound of his voice, even when I didn't understand every word he was saying.

Each time we sat down for a meal, we'd go around to say what we were grateful for. Whenever it was his turn, my future father-in-law could never get through it. As soon as the first word came out, the tears started flowing because he loved his family so, so much. And how they loved him.

His love for family spoke to me, moved me, and felt aligned with my soul. Seeing that familial love—how he was with his wife and children—made my own love for Alejandro even more intense. I knew that our wedding picture and the pictures of our children would be in that briefcase someday. He would be showing *our* pictures to strangers and tearing up about us.

My affection for this family grew by the day. I didn't want our time together to end.

Celebratory Dinner

Every day, we passed by a lovely little restaurant called La Capilla in the neighborhood where we were staying. It was in the center of the historic district, connected by one wall to the gorgeous Parroquia, the seventeenth-century cathedral. The dining area was open air and, though it was ancient, it was spectacular—very old-world, so romantic and glorious. When the sun set, they'd light dozens of candles in the most beautiful wrought-iron candelabras that stood tall in the open windows. Those beeswax candles dripped in elegant pools on the floor. Spanish guitar music wafted out onto the street. It was on my bucket list to eat there, so to celebrate on my last day of classes, we made a reservation at La Capilla at sunset. I was sure it'd be worth the wait and a perfect way to close our adventure together.

I'd been learning a lot about patience over the last few months. We'd get engaged when my annulment papers were signed, sealed, and delivered. But the wheels of government were turning slowly. I had no idea when they might finally arrive.

On that last day of school, I was excited for our special dinner. My future mother-in-law said, *"Ve ducharte y vistete."* ("Go take a shower and get dressed.")

I said, "No, it's okay, I'm fine. Let's just go!" But we weren't leaving just yet. Alejandro's dad mixed palomas, a delicious cocktail made with tequila, lime juice, and grapefruit. He sat me down and handed me one, then showed me a video Alejandro had sent. It was a really sweet montage of pictures of us accompanied by Nat King Cole's song, "L-O-V-E," *"L is for the way you look at me . . ."* along with a wonderful letter Alejandro had sent, saying how proud he was of me for finishing my course and how special it made him feel that I wanted to learn his first language in order to communicate with his family. I felt so cared for, so loved.

Then we headed out for our dinner together.

At La Capilla, his mom and I basked in the glow of all those candles as a Spanish guitarist played. We ordered a delicious meal, then my mother-in-law excused herself for the restroom. As she walked away I noticed a mariachi band was ascending ancient stairs to play for the guests. I looked around thinking, *Oh, I hope she hurries back! She loves mariachi.* I was so excited!

I noticed one of the mariachi members was wearing white. Everyone else was wearing black. I assumed he must be the lead singer of the group. Also he was holding his hat in front of his face. Was he holding on to it so it wouldn't blow away in the breeze? We were outside, after all. Then the band started walking toward our table. I thought, "This is great! Where is Alejandro's mom?" Then suddenly that white hat popped up—that "band member" was Alejandro! As the group played, he dropped down on one knee and proposed. I of course said *yes*!

Initially I was in complete shock. What was he doing here? He was supposed to be in Miami. It was the most surprising, sweetest moment. My father-in-law captured the whole thing on video. As my mother-in-law walked over, beaming, I said, "You should have made me take that shower." After all, I hadn't seen Alejandro for weeks. If I'd had a clue this would happen, I would have dressed up a bit. But that didn't matter. It was wonderful. Knowing that my future in-laws had been in on this surprise with Alejandro made my joy that much greater.

Officially Family

We married in San Miguel de Allende a year later in a centuries-old church called Templo de San Francisco. It was a traditional Mexican wedding and, funnily enough, it was a bit like a parade back home in Louisiana—a joyful troupe of laughing, smiling celebrants. While our guests walked with us from the church to the reception, a burro (donkey) walked along with us, carrying sipping tequila in carved out cucumbers in baskets on his back. It was quite a celebration! There were even giant puppets called *mojigangas*, a tradition brought to San Miguel from Spain in the 1600s, that joined us on the journey from the church to the reception.

Alejandro and I rode through town in a carriage with our procession as a mariachi band played, churros were eaten, tequila was tasted, puppets danced, and guests laughed and sang. All the people came out of the shops and their homes lining the streets, cheering us on and wishing us well. It was quite spectacular, and a moment I will never forget. We had all our family with us. It was the sweetest sendoff for our life together.

I'd gone to Mexico to learn how to communicate with my future in-laws. How could I have known that our time together there would make us family even before I married my husband? I got to know them not just through words but through the intimate gestures, habits, and laughter that you see when you wake up to someone. It showed me their true character. By the end of the trip the three of us had formed a special bond, so much that when my husband got there, I was a little like, "Hm. Do I have to share them with you?" I'd enjoyed all their attention! I was so glad we'd had that time together to form our own relationships. It was a gift I hadn't even known to ask for. And that relationship grew over time.

Soul Ache

Years later, in fall 2015, we received a phone call that would change every part of our lives forever. My father-in-law (Juan Manuel Gomez Fernandez) and Alejandro's brother (Juan Manuel Gomez Monteverde) had been kidnapped outside their hometown in Mexico.

Days passed. Still, they were not released. Then we learned the horrible truth. They were gone.

It was devastating. There are no words to describe the grief. It is hard enough when you have to mourn one loved one in these unimaginable circumstances, but to mourn two? How could we bear it?

Denial is one of the stages of grief. When we found out about the kidnapping, my first thought was that those who did this would fall in love with my father-in-law. *He is going to find a way to charm them, and they are going to let him go.* How could anyone ever harm someone so full of life and love? It seemed incomprehensible.

> May love be what you remember most.
>
> *Darcie Sims*

While I reeled from the news, I knew my place was to be there for Alejandro, both of us mourning while keeping the truth from our kids because we didn't feel they were old enough to understand what happened.

The grief and the pain felt like we were carrying a building on our shoulders. It was the greatest weight I ever experienced, pulling me down all the time. Losing them changed everything. I was not the same person. Little things—everything that used to feel important—material things, jobs, goals—suddenly were less important. Sitting with the pain was important but it was difficult to do.

I was struck by what I read in *The Most Important Thing* by Howard Marks. He wrote about the transformation that can result from tragedy or deep difficulty. Pain can be both a challenge and an opportunity. This quote stuck with me:

How we respond [to suffering] is important. Do we search for a quick solution, quick answer or someone to save us? Or do we settle into those moments and meet ourselves?[3]

I had to let go of what wasn't serving me anymore—thoughts, behaviors, even things—to be transformed by these events. Otherwise, I'd be swallowed whole. I knew in my soul that there must be blessings yet to be perceived; otherwise it was all unbearable.

Faith Put to the Test

In tragedy, faith is truly put to the test. Honestly, that was the most difficult thing in all of this for me. Suffering had sent me to my knees in prayer so many times. Now it was hard to pray. I initially felt betrayed by God. I tried and tried, but I could not understand. Remember how Jesus called to God on the cross, "Why have you forsaken me?" (Matthew 27:46). *Forsaken* felt like the right word. How could God let darkness snuff out such a joyful, pure heart? That was really, really hard.

My family and I were still going through the motions of going to church on Sundays, but it was as if we went under obligation. There was no joy in it for me. I was showing up but keeping my heart from being open in a way. I'd agreed to host a Catholic conference in Florida, and honoring that "obligation" turned out to be an amazing mercy for me. See, even though I'd been a practicing Catholic for years, I never had a devotion to Mary, partly because of my experience with the nondenominational Protestant kind of faith. I pray to Jesus, going straight to him, not "bothering" with the saints. I met a priest at this conference named Father Michael Gaitley. He'd written a book called *33 Days to Morning Glory*, a daily devotional with readings from the Gospels about Mary. The point is to avail yourself Mary's assistance in going before her Son, Jesus.

As the host of the conference, sitting on the side, listening to him talk, I sensed a breakthrough idea was forming. Alejandro was back in the hotel room, but I knew he needed to hear this, so I set up a meeting with Father Gaitley. Alejandro and I were both still in a place of struggle, not understanding why God allowed such a tragedy. With Father Gaitley's insights about Mary, I saw that this was an opportunity. I didn't feel comfortable going straight to God right then, but Mary, the mother of God? She's a mother too, and a daughter, and a wife. I relate to her; she felt safe to me right then and maybe she could comfort me. I thought I could talk to her. For the very first time in my life that made sense.

So, for the next month, I prayed to Mary, the mother of God, and poured out my heart. That was a turning point for me. Talking with her helped bring me back into a full relationship with her Son, Jesus. I began to see the grace and the mercies in my life in a new way. Mary brought me back to Jesus.

For me, Mary was a lifeline to my faith. Find something that will anchor you to yours. Maybe it will be a book or piece of music that sustains you—maybe all of the above. The important thing is not to let the flame of your faith be extinguished; it is the only thing that can keep some of us going through the most difficult times.

A Window in My Soul

Once that healing process started, a window opened in my soul.

That process, the whole thing, challenged me to look at life in a new way. We know in a real way that life is short. I started prioritizing time together as a family and one-on-one relationships. I make time to get outside of my own head and see the bigger picture and appreciate the gifts of life. One of my favorite things is to take my family and go to the ocean. The expanse of it, the sound of the waves rhythmically crashing on the shore, reminds us of our little place in this great expanse of time that is life.

We decided to focus on the beauty of my father- and brother-in-law's lives, how they lived instead of how they left us. I feel their presence daily. I sense it in our lives, in a strong, powerful way. My husband does too. We feel like they are active participants in our lives. In a way, we are probably closer to them now than when they were on the earth with us physically.

At this point in our lives, we decided to focus on what John Green described so well:

> Grief does not change you. . . . It reveals you. And herein lies the gift that cannot die. It changes the course of your life forever. If you allow yourself the chance to feel it for as long as you need to even if it is for the rest of your life, you will be guided by it. You will become someone it would have been impossible for you to be, and in this way your loved one lives on, in you.[4]

Going through grief and loss wasn't what I would have chosen. None of us would intentionally choose pain and suffering for ourselves. But we each suffer. And we learn that good things emerge from hard things. It's a process. You may have experienced this in your own life. Loss has a way of teaching you what you didn't want to learn.

Granted, growing into my own soul reshape with this didn't happen overnight. It happened through sitting with the pain, not deflecting it, and allowing grace to come in and progress to occur. There's no way it could have happened if we'd just moved on and not tried to seek out a greater understanding. Difficult things happen, but if we look for it, we can find a new way of walking through life—a true transformation in the best possible way.

Grief can be excruciating. Waves of it can knock you off your feet. It's intense on a physical, mental, and spiritual level. What's beautiful is that in such moments of overwhelm, we have an opportunity to be transformed. There's tremendous grace in such times. Just when we find the limits of what we can stand, breakthrough happens. I've experienced such grace and have actively received it. I received that grace with my body, mind, and soul.

So much good has shown up for the family—and is still coming out of it. We are closer and our joys all the sweeter because of the things we've weathered together.

Never in my wildest dreams would I have imagined our family could suffer such a tragedy. I wouldn't wish it on anyone. Going through it hurt—sometimes it still hurts. But having lived through it, I can finally see the blessings in it. It forced myself and my husband to view life as a one-chance opportunity, realizing how short it really is. It is precious, and we don't want to take a moment for granted. We will not allow circumstances to define us and keep us from truly living. We want to live in gratitude, awareness, and intent, not habit. We want to make life something beautiful. We want to be purposeful in how we walk through this life. We want a life we love, that my father- and brother-in-law would be proud of.

Practices that Shape My Soul

We have all suffered trauma to one degree or another. Suffering is part of the human condition. I'm learning that, if you let it, suffering can help reshape your soul in positive ways.

Looking back, I see how the routines of that special summer in Mexico fortified me. In the last few years I've established new routines to help center me and actively reshape my soul. I'd like to share some of my practices with you in hopes that they'll prepare you for the inevitable bumps and bruises life doles out.

Soul on Fire

Going through that grieving process forced me to think deeply about purpose, joy, and the choices we make every day. We're each given just one life. We get to choose whether we live frantic, over-scheduled lives or prioritized lives. We choose whether we're going to compare our lives to others' or if we are going to set our own path and fill our days with the people we love, building relationships and creating a life of adventure.

From the start of our relationship, Alejandro and I resolved to build a big life together full of meaningful moments focused on family. Tragedy deepened our commitment to actively create a world that reflects God's glory. Life is short, so our mantra has become, *Live in a way that sets your soul on fire.* It's what his father and brother would have wanted.

Only you can recognize what makes you feel truly alive. When I became a mom for the first time, everyone would ask me how it felt. I described it as a joy I felt in the depths of my soul. Funny, I was connecting to my soul even then. When you are doing something and you hear that little voice in your head that says, "Yeah, that's it!" your heart gets warm and you don't even know how to express the joy and excitement you feel. Do more of that! Do more of what sets your soul on fire.

A soul reshape starts with taking inventory of the way you move about the world. Are you seeking joy? Are you fulfilling your purpose? Or are you going through the motions of life because it's easy and is what you know? Are you afraid to jump into something new and take a risk? Do you feel a joy in the depths of your soul? What is the point of doing anything if our souls are not alive? Close your eyes and imagine the best possible version of yourself. That's who you really are. Let go of any part of you that doesn't align with this. It is important to be fearless in what sets your soul on fire.

Being in tune with your own soul brings a greater connection to humanity as we remember that each of us is alive for a greater purpose than ourselves. It's a reminder of the dignity of each and every soul.

Nature's Soul Connection

One day I was walking in my neighborhood and came upon a tree marked with a heart-shaped knot. Nature had birthed this knot, but it was so perfectly shaped that it seemed like an artisan had carved the heart out with a tool! I took a photo and sent it to one of my friends. Her response was, "That's God's daily gift." I love that idea because what she said is true. God gives us gifts every day; we just have to be *aware* enough to see it. To acknowledge it. And be appreciative. We have to be present in our lives to stop and see the beauty that is all around us. When we're as present and attentive as young children, we'll see beauty in nature, in travel, in people; it really is everywhere.

When I spend time outdoors, I feel a strong sense of gratitude. It bubbles up from inside me. Just seeing God's creation brings a deep peace. Having discovered how centered and whole it makes me feel, I've made a point to reshape my schedule. I spend time outside as much as possible every day, and I love to hike on the mountain behind my house. My kids love running through the sprinkler as they end a summer day, and we ride bikes as a family to our favorite local restaurant. I love foraging for wild branches and flowers to create beautiful displays on our dining table. An evening walk with my husband is good for my soul but also keeps me connected to him. Being outside always makes me feel grounded—when I am barefoot it's even better—and it daily reshapes my perspective. I see God's glory reflected in everything before my eyes.

When you see the beauty around you and allow yourself to feel that overwhelming sense of gratitude, peace, and wholeness, you will feel truly alive. Seeking out what's naturally beautiful taps into our soulfulness, into the full spectrum of who we are. It's easy to be jaded by the cynicism and negativity in our day-to-day lives. We combat this when we're actively observant of the beauty of our surroundings. Again, it's a choice that's ours alone.

Create a Morning Quiet-Time Ritual

Getting up just an hour earlier than my family wakes up allows me some quiet, soul-centering time. It makes me feel grounded and centered. When I miss out on that time, I'm off-center and more easily annoyed and frazzled. Here's what it looks like for me. When my alarm goes off, I open my eyes and say thank you to God. That's huge for me—to make the very first act of my day an act of gratitude to God. While I am drinking my first liter of water based on the SWW Method, I write in my gratitude journal to put me in the right mindset. At this point the house is quiet— the kids are still sleeping. So, I go downstairs, prepare a hot cup of water with lemon, and light a candle. I sit still and breathe. I keep inspirational books next to my chair so I can center my mind if necessary. I'll pray and meditate, talking to God and listening to God's prompts. This time is really about allowing the peace of God to permeate my soul. It's a routine and practice that truly sets the tone for my day and ultimately for my life. I empty out all my worries, fears, and anxiety and give God the space to come in and work.

How Has Loss Shaped Your Life?

Take a moment to think about how a specific loss has shaped your own life experience. The loss could be a person, a relationship, a career, or a tragic experience. Does that loss feel painful even now? Why or why not?

If you need a soul reshape, reflect on your life. What is your reason for a soul reshape? Make a list of the times when you feel that warmth in your soul that I shared about. What are you doing when you feel that? That's what you need to do more of. Repairing your soul will happen naturally when you begin to make movement in small areas. When you focus on the shape of your mind, the quality of your thoughts, the practices you put in place, all while holding yourself accountable, you will eventually lead yourself to a full soul reshape.

How do you tap into soulfulness? When do you feel like your soul is set free? Spending time with loved ones? Taking in nature? Looking at the expanse of the ocean? Doing a hobby you love? Working on a passion project?

—————— RESHAPE WRAP-UP ——————

Understand—for yourself and the condition of your soul—the spiritual connection you have to the world and the life you are living. I believe the soul is a combination of three things: intelligence, reason, and passion. Is your soul alive, or does it need a reshape?

There is purpose in our most painful moments. The painful moments are defining. God does not let any of it go to waste, though. It is up to us how we will respond to the difficulties that inevitably impact our lives. All pain is not equal, but how we respond to it begins with conditioning our mindset.

Invest in your spiritual self. Seek out your greater purpose. Curating a beautiful life includes creating space for the activities and feelings that set your soul on fire.

RESHAPE MOVES —————————————————

1. What sets your soul on fire? When do you feel the most fulfilled and living out your true calling? In my own life, I find that my purpose and feeling joy down deep is always connected to when I am serving others in some way.

2. Find other people who share similar interests and whom you can share significant moments with. We are not meant to walk through life alone. The bonds you build with your closest loved ones bring peace and feed your soul regularly.

3. If you feel like you need a soul reshape, begin to change small things with your activities, how you spend your time, what you think about and focus on. How much time do we all spend really thinking about this? Life moves so quickly; we need to show our soul some love on a regular basis.

CHAPTER 7

RESHAPE YOUR REST

The Key to Experiencing

Next-Level Wellness

The more you thank Life, the more Life
will give you to be thankful for.

LOUISE HAY

I'd enjoyed sweet "mandatory" siestas in Mexico with my in-laws—and those might have been the first real, disciplined rest I'd ever experienced. Although I was on "hiatus" (which literally means *rest*) from work, my personality craved productivity, so I'd insisted on using the time to learn a new language. Little did I know that in that pursuit, I'd also learn the rhythm of rest.

The concept of rest was new to me. I didn't really know the value of rest before. After all, my mother seemed to never rest. Then I began to struggle with sleep, mostly because of pain that resulted from an earlier car accident. I also had some daily habits that kept me from sleeping well. At night I wrestled with the sheets, trying to fall sleep. I'd wake up frequently during the night. Then, when the alarm rang, I had trouble properly waking up because I hadn't gotten enough rest. When my kids were young, sleep schedules got more erratic. I was often running on fumes.

I suffered from lack of sleep for years.

Then I had a life-changing encounter with "The Sleep Doctor," Dr. Michael Breus. We were both on the set of the Hallmark Channel's *Home and Family*, where I was promoting a yearly child safety event I started after I had my children. I'd become an advocate for car-seat safety and became a certified car-seat technician. Dr. Breus was talking about the new concept of chronotypes, which he talks about in his book *The Power of When*. When I heard him referred to as a "Sleep Doctor" I thought, *That's exactly what I need!* I cornered him and told him about my struggles with insomnia. I learned more about sleep from him in five minutes than I'd heard in my entire life. That was the start of a friendship that's been an absolutely wonderful life change for me. I'll let him tell you about that in his own words.

Meet the Expert: Dr. Michael Breus

I met Ali on the set of a national media program. Ali expressed that she was anxious about her lack of sleep. I assured her that what she was feeling was completely normal. When people struggle with sleep, it naturally makes them feel anxious. Feeling out of control provokes anxiety—and a lack of sleep exacerbates that feeling. It's a vicious cycle. A good remedy for sleep anxiety is information. When you know more about the science of sleep, you start to feel some measure of control. And that lessens your anxiety, which makes sleep easier to come by. It's almost a sleep hack.

Based on our initial meeting, I knew Ali was doing a lot of the right things: eating well, exercising, not doing drugs. That said, she was dealing with pain issues that interrupted her sleep. Once I pointed her in the direction of some ways to get that pain addressed, we addressed her sleep environment. I gave her some things to do to make that environment more conducive to good sleep. Were her mattress, sheets, and pillows working well for her, or did they need replacing? And was her room the optimal temperature?

Soon Ali had made some significant changes that helped her get higher quality, more consistent sleep. She'll be the first to tell you it made a huge difference in her quality of life.

If you're dealing with sleep issues like Ali was, I recommend you start with these five simple steps, just like Ali did.

1. **Wake up at one time, every day.** Waking up at the same time each day—and that includes weekends—trains your body to turn off the hormones that regulate sleep at the same time each day.

2. **Don't take any caffeine after two in the afternoon.** Caffeine stays in your system for six to eight hours. If you're aiming to go to sleep between ten and midnight, you need to be off it by two.

3. **Limit alcohol use.** Two glasses of wine have been shown to increase sleep by fifteen minutes, but after *three*, the benefits reverse. Three drinks are actually *detrimental* to sleep. Also, give your alcohol *three* hours to digest before sleep. For example, if you're aiming to go to sleep at ten o'clock, that last drink should stop at seven. (Pro-tip: drink one glass of water in between each alcoholic beverage for optimal hydration to offset the dehydrating effects of alcohol.)

4. **Exercise.** I'm a huge advocate for exercise, getting your heart rate up and muscles moving. That said, exercise ramps up energy, so it's smart to get that workout in *four* hours before bed, at minimum. If at all possible, get that workout in during the morning. That's best. The body's core body temperature drops naturally at around 10:30 p.m., releasing melatonin, the body's natural sleep hormone. If you've elevated your body temperature through a workout, the melatonin isn't going to kick in.

5. **Finally, how you wake determines how you sleep.** To truly turn off the melatonin faucet, upon waking, don't

just hit the snooze alarm. Sit up and swing your legs on the side of the bed. Take *fifteen* deep breaths. Drink *fifteen* ounces of water to rehydrate what the body has lost overnight. Then spend *fifteen* minutes outside in the sun every morning within the first half hour of rising. It might sound nuts, but I highly recommend bare feet in the morning—it's literally grounding. Again, exposure to sunshine turns off the melatonin faucet and helps cut through brain fog.

Finally, for better sleep, I prescribe unconditional love, like the love of a dog or cat. Love works wonders for body, mind, and soul!

I started experiencing consistent, restorative sleep for the first time in years once I began implementing Dr. Breus's suggestions. I found that by following his advice, I was waking up refreshed. I had new energy. My mental and physical health and performance improved in ways I never could have imagined. The rest I was getting actually took me to a whole new level of wellness!

The improvements piqued my interest in sleep, and I sensed that if I had access to more information, I could up-level my performance in other areas as well.

That's when I discovered one of my favorite tools in my wellness toolbox: the Oura Ring. It's a very lightweight ring that I wear on my left hand. This little gadget is the most comprehensive sleep tracker on the market. It tracks my biology at all times. The biofeedback is then translated into data I can read on my phone. Every morning, I'm getting customized information. The ring calculates my sleep score and suggests optimal times for me to exercise, eat, and take a break. It's been so valuable to me in learning about what works for my sleep and my body. (While they do not provide the comprehensive data that the Oura Ring provides, the Apple Watch and Fitbit have sleep-tracking features as well.)

But even before I got this ring, Dr. Breus challenged me to track what he called my "sleep hygiene" in a journal. I wrote down when I went to bed, what I did in bed (read, watch TV, snack, etc.), approximately how long it took me to go to sleep, and then I wrote down if I woke up in the night and if so, how many times—and I kept a tally of how many hours I slept. This journal helped me identify patterns—the good ones and the ones that were keeping me from falling asleep and staying asleep.

Now that I have my Oura Ring, I check it every morning. I know myself and how competitive I can get with myself, so this holds me accountable for making good choices that day. It also helps me give myself grace if the previous night's rating was fairly low. I know from experience that the higher the quality of my sleep, the better I feel—and the better I feel, the more I can accomplish. So, if I had a low-quality sleep rating, I might put off a super challenging task for a day until I can do it on a full tank, so to speak.

Rest 2.0

Sleep is restful, but make no mistake: rest is more than sleep. It's a mindset. As a type-A overachiever, if I'm not mindful of rest, I will exhaust myself.

Rest, for me, has become about establishing healthy routines, rhythms, and boundaries. One of my favorites is the daily rhythm of waking up each morning early enough to spend time in meditation and prayer.

I mentioned earlier that I've been practicing meditation for many years now. For me, meditating is an opportunity to experience a different way of perceiving my life. I sit quietly and allow myself the space to just be. I tap into my most essential self—my soul—letting the rest fall away. I sit in silence and, with each breath, empty out all my worries, fears, insecurities, and running to-do lists, asking God for what my heart and soul desires in as much detail as possible, trusting him to fill me back up with what I need to move forward into my day.

Meditation is many things. It's prayer, breath, wondering, dreaming, curiosity, writing, reading, movement, stretching, manifesting, curating in my mind, practicing, and slowly seeing all of it show up.

Before bed it allows me to let go of the day's stress and worries, puts me a relaxed state, and can actually induce melatonin production, helping me get to sleep faster.

The Best Rest

I have a "no guilt" approach to self-care. I don't feel guilty, for instance, about taking good care of my skin. My mom taught me that if I don't take care of myself, no one else will. That truth—especially coming from her—was a huge gift. That said, I struggled for many years to put that kind of self-care into practice when it came to rest.

I've learned that to be well rested I need to be kind to myself. I try *not* to multitask when I can. At other times, especially when the kids are home, I am tending to their needs, helping with homework, cooking dinner, running them around, taking the dog for a walk, and finishing up my day's work. I allow myself time each week to be "off"—typically that's Sunday, but sometimes it's a different day. I also look at my calendar every year and consciously schedule pockets of time when I can rest and recharge.

Taking time for meditation in the morning completely changes the course of my day. If I do my morning routine of waking up early for a time of gratitude, quiet, water, lemon water, green juice, coffee, and meditation, then a workout—it's "Look out, world!" I'm rested and energized for the whole day.

If like me you've wrestled with overdoing it, I hope you'll try some of the things in this chapter. You deserve better rest. Implementing rest and quality sleep in your life has been on the top-five list of every health expert I have spoken to. It is an action you can take personally to restore your health. By sleeping better and having a mindset of rest, you will experience next-level wellness—and, if you're like me, you'll find you'll never want to go back.

In practicing this reshape, I'm careful about my social media use. I have a love-hate relationship with all forms of social media. I do enjoy sharing snippets of my life with friends, but I don't like the feeling that I *have* to share. Unfortunately, the entertainment business requires constant engagement—I get or lose jobs based on it. I do love listening to experts and finding new, usable information that I can apply or share with our RE/SHAPE community. Being inspired by design or reading a quote that unexpectedly turns a light on in my mind is a great use of social media for me. It's also a good way to stay caught up with friends I don't see as often as I'd like.

That said, for my own mental well-being, I choose not to be on social media constantly. And I have a teenage daughter for whom I want to model healthy social media habits. My daughter is fifteen and does not have her own cell phone or use social media. It's a decision we made as parents to protect her self-esteem, confidence, and mental well-being. I have very strong feelings about the effects of social media on children. It affects adults as well. The only difference is that adults can manage the effects slightly more. So for me, I post and then I am out. I respond and look at comments the next day at a specific time: before I prepare dinner. I may scroll for a bit to see what's happening. I do not log on to the app mindlessly when I have a spare moment because I know habitual scrolling is bad for me emotionally and mentally. I remind myself that everything *looks* perfect on socials, but looks can be deceiving. I also remind myself that a person is worth more than the number of followers or the soulless validation of a checkmark by the name. My self-worth does not come from a screen on my laptop or in my hand. If I start to feel self-doubt creeping in when I'm on social media, I log off immediately. Life is too short to waste it in mental head games or comparisons. If something isn't serving you, you're allowed to let go of it. Release it for now or forever, whatever works for you. You know you and you need to protect you from anything that could deter you from keeping a healthy mindset and impacting your overall well-being.

I don't know about you, but as I have gotten older, my body needs more time to recover. My whole body—not just my back or my legs but my brain too. Resting and recovery is certainly an art. It's creating an ideal space and implementing reinforcements that work for you: the bedding, lighting, music, drinks that settle you, and diffusing soothing oil aromas. Routines around sleep and giving your body rest only help you maintain an optimal level of restorative time for your body, all the way down to the cellular level. I mean, if you are going to spend time resting or sleeping for eight hours of your life every day, don't you want to maximize the benefit? I know we would want to with anything else we spend that amount of time on.

Whether you think you sleep well or have some trouble like me, once you assess your sleep patterns and figure out what type of sleeper you are, you can begin the exciting work of a customized reshape around your rest, all of which will enhance your life and allow you to begin your day feeling like you are running your world and your world is not running you.

Gratitude

My friend Roma Downey sat down to talk with me about how she starts her day. I love that she says "thank you" aloud as each foot hits the floor every morning. It turns out Roma is onto something. This is a sort of bio-hack, according to UCLA's Mindful Awareness Research Center. Having an attitude of gratitude literally affects the central nervous system, changing your molecular structure, keeping us "healthier and happier."[5]

—————— RESHAPE WRAP-UP ——————

By creating an optimal sleep environment, better sleep is achievable. Assess your sleeping environment, reshape your routine, and make the necessary updates to give yourself the proper sleep setting.

Rest isn't just about sleep. It's providing the time necessary for your entire body to rebuild itself at the cellular level. Resting brings peace to your body and restores your mind, your digestion, blood pressure, the list goes on. Prioritize your rest every day. Don't forget, much of the world rests on Sundays and often takes a siesta during weekdays.

There is power generated for your life by daily sleep and rest cycles. Figure out what kind of sleeper you are based on Dr. Breus's test. Only then can you know how to best serve yourself and create a proper routine.

RESHAPE MOVES ———————————————

1. If sleep is an issue for you, track your sleep hygiene for a week or two. Record when you lie down, what you do before sleep (read, watch TV, snack), approximately how long it takes you to go to sleep, and how many times you wake. Keep a record of how many hours of sleep you get. You'll begin to see patterns. The Oura Ring is great for this.

2. Try Dr. Breus's tips:
   - Wake up at the same time daily.
   - Limit caffeine to mornings, making sure to have that last cup no later than 2:00 p.m.
   - Limit alcohol use and be sure your final drink is finished three hours before bed.

3. Promote an environment of relaxation a few hours before heading to bed. Dim the lights, quiet down, put all your electronics on night mode.

CHAPTER 8

RESHAPE YOUR BEAUTY

The LA Angel Who Taught Me to Fly

Beauty is how you feel inside, and it reflects
in your eyes. It is not something physical.

SOPHIA LOREN

When I first moved to LA all those years ago, I enjoyed monthly facials at an exclusive place in Bel Air called Vera's Retreat in the Glen. It was one of the amazing perks of being Miss USA. The owner of the place was a wonderful woman named Vera Brown, and she became for me the gold standard of what beauty looks like.

Vera was an angel, always helping others and genuinely connecting with people. I was so drawn to her heart and her beautiful spirit. She was in her seventies when we met. To me, she epitomized old Hollywood. She ran around with Frank Sinatra and that set. She was legendary. At her salon in those days, you might run into Nicole Kidman, Jane Seymore, or Whitney Houston in the lobby. That's the kind of clientele who sought out her services.

But Vera didn't hoard her talent. She worked with glamorous stars and the rich and famous, but she also served women in shelters and juvenile halls. She believed every woman is beautiful. Happily for me, Vera took me under her wing when I had just moved to Los Angeles and became my protector, my angel, and she taught me the standard by which I measure beauty.

I'd grown up in the business of beauty, with my mom's beauty salon next door to my house. My entire young life I saw women coming in to get their hair done and to share what was going on in their lives. They always walked out feeling a little more glamorous, more put together, more confident, even with a little more sass in their walk. They were glowing when they walked out of my mom's salon. So I felt comfortable in Vera's salon. But I had a lot to learn from her.

Beauty from the Inside Out

I remember washing my face with Vera's famous aloe vera cleanser as Vera stood close by. As I scrubbed my makeup off in the same lackadaisical way I did every day, Vera stopped me. She stood next to me at the sink and said, "Try it like this." She lathered some cleanser in her hand with a little water, then rubbed it in small circles all around her face. Looking at her own reflection in the mirror she smiled and said, "I am beautiful and I am enough. I treat myself with kindness."

Vera took my concept of beauty to a whole new level.

Love in Action

Soon after we met, Vera invited me to her lake house in Lake Sherwood where she was doing a day retreat for the girls from an institution called MacLaren Hall. She wanted to know if I would help. I was new to town and didn't know the area very well, but I agreed right away. Whatever she was doing, I wanted to be a part of it.

I learned that MacLaren Hall served girls who were in the state system. Vera wanted to help these girls, and she did that by offering what she was good at. She was wonderful at being present with them. She told them how beautiful and perfect they were. She taught them how to care for their skin and hair. Some had never received that kind of attention. She'd hand them a mirror and say in her sweet voice, "Look at yourself! Aren't you lovely? Say, 'Hi! How are you today? You are so amazing! I love you so much!'" She taught them how to love themselves through self-care. She believed that self-love is the greatest healer of trauma. I saw the truth of this firsthand. It was a beautiful thing to witness.

That's how we truly connected through serving others. What really impressed me was that Vera treated the girls at MacLaren just as she did all the beautiful and glamorous stars who came through her spa: with love and respect.

Helping Vera with the girls from MacLaren Hall got me hooked. I would go with Vera just about everywhere after that. She gave workshops and clinics. She gave free facials, haircuts, makeup lessons, and manicures to girls struggling with abuse, cancer, physical handicaps, and poverty.

I also served alongside Vera with People Assisting the Homeless (PATH), an organization in California that is dedicated to helping people find permanent housing and that provides case management, medical care, employment training, and other services to maintain stability. Vera provided a beauty salon where women and girls could get their hair done and receive spa services. PATH also helped women clear their records in the court system: outstanding tickets, violations, and other issues. They could even learn a trade there. Vicky, a woman who went through PATH with her children, studied hair and makeup. Vera saw her heart and connected with her. Vera put Vicky through cosmetology school and, when she graduated, offered her a job at Vera's day spa in Bel Air. Vera paid for her to have her smile fixed and set up her apartment. She was a lot of people's angel, it seems.

Seeing Vera love people so well made me respect her so much. I felt grateful to be a part of her life and to witness her in action. She was old enough to be my grandmother. I loved her like one too. I was always holding her hand, hugging her, or rubbing her arm. Somehow I knew that even though she looked like a million bucks, she wasn't long for this world. She had many health issues. She had spine issues. She had foot issues. She never complained, but she had a team of people who helped her. She took good care of herself. I remember seeing lots of herbs, supplements, and gadgets at her house. I felt an urge to protect her and take care of her. Anytime we were together, I would open the door for her. I'd hold her purse and take her arm to steady her wherever we went. I helped her to her car, put her in, and closed the door for her. It was an honor to stand next to her; maybe I was hoping some of her goodness would rub off on me.

She passed more than ten years ago, and I am so grateful she was able to meet my baby daughter Estela before she passed. Vera was my family in Los Angeles, and the fact that she'd taken me under her wing was such a gift. To this day I still have some of her products. Seeing them reminds me of her, of her love, of her spirit.

> Beauty is not in the face; beauty is a light in the heart.
>
> *Khalil Gibran*

Vera was the next-level version of what I'd seen growing up in my mom's beauty shop—she showed me that beauty and mindset are inextricably linked. She helped me discover that when you tap into a healthy mindset, something beautiful shines through. She taught me never to judge anyone, to always look past their exterior and search for their heart and really *see* them.

Friends Who Feel Like Sunshine

I wanted to be with Vera as much as I could because she inspired me. I felt like she was a gift sent from God to guide me at this time in my life. From her I discovered that I have a choice: I choose to surround myself with people who raise my sights and inspire me to live my best life!

The people you surround yourself with should feel like sunshine. When you are around them, you feel their light and it warms your soul. I have so many friends, men and women, in my life who seem to have light exuding from them. They look at the world in broad, colorful strokes, not focusing on the little things that don't really matter or serve us. They are the kind of people who see your superpowers. They see you for who you really are, in the depths of you—the places you don't always show the world. They are the kind of people who lift you up. After I've been around these friends, I am not kidding, my body feels electrified. I feel hopeful and positive. Edit your friends—and I don't mean that in a mean way. We are not in high school anymore. We don't have to be on the playground with the mean girl. There are some people in our lives, maybe friends or even family, who are toxic. You can still be kind, but protect yourself or limit your time with them.

Have you ever heard the saying, "Show me your friends and I will show you your future"? This is truer than you may realize. Many areas of our lives are defined by our environment and the people in it. Friendships are an ongoing reshape in most of our lives. Some people are there for a season, some people are there for a purpose, and some are there for a lifetime. Everyone holds a different value for your life. Approaching your relationships with this in mind can help you evaluate how to reshape this area of your life.

The world needs more women who lift each other up—women who don't look to material things to fill up what may be missing in their lives. That mindset can be summed up with one word: *celebrate*. Celebrate what's good in others' lives; don't compare. When you see good happening in another woman's life, choose to celebrate it—even serving alongside them if you want to.

If we truly acknowledge that we were all created with individual gifts and a specific purpose, it helps to release any type of comparison. You can go live your life, experience the ups and downs, and recognize along the way that you are doing you. No one else has lived your life, has had your experiences or your history. And you have not had theirs. The most in-your-face place for feelings of comparison to creep in is through social media. Again, use social media for what you want; be in control of your mind and emotions. Comparing, coveting, or thinking less of yourself based on a produced version of someone else's life is hardly a way to live. Just do you and assume other women are doing their best to do the same. This creates an internal beauty that shines through.

Sharing Is Beautiful

Vera's example also showed me how sharing from your heart is beauty, plain and simple. Whatever your gift is, find a way to share it! God gave us our gifts for a reason, and it is our responsibility to share those gifts. My daughter was given a beautiful voice as a gift, and sometimes when she is asked to sing she pushes back, especially now that she is in her teenage years. I always remind her that her voice is her gift from God and it is her responsibility to share that gift to bring joy to others.

As I've shared, I like to see myself as a student of life, a voracious learner, always welcoming personal growth. When it comes to wellness, I am curious, an explorer. I am grateful for the opportunities I have had to try new products and modalities for healing—and sharing what I have learned. I feel like in a small way I'm living out the legacy of my angel, Vera, when I share that a little bit of her light is shining through me.

First Inner Beauty, Then Outer Beauty

Now, after you've gotten your internal beauty mindset in shape, it's time to address the outside. I've had the most amazing opportunity over the years in the entertainment business to work with the best hair and makeup artists, top stylists, fitness experts, and treatment providers. I have learned and absorbed so much information from these professionals, including tips, techniques, and trade secrets that I have learned to customize and put to use for what works for me. And again, I love sharing what I've learned, whether it's about that five-minute makeup application that I can take from day to night or about styling my wardrobe in such a way that I can pair designer pieces with bargain finds. Here are my best tips for outer beauty.

Skin and Makeup

I'm particular with my skincare routine. I think I developed this interest while selling skincare in my mom's salon to put myself through college. Ladies would come into the salon, and after their hair was done, I would finish their look with a new makeup application, testing shades that were new to them or applying them in ways they had never tried. Seeing the women walk out feeling their best with fresh hair and makeup, I was hooked.

I think by now I have tried every skincare and makeup product available, whether it's been gifted to me, a makeup artist has used it on me, or I have found it on my own search for new products. One thing is for sure: creating a routine for your skin and sticking to it will give a big payoff in the long run. I often receive compliments on my skin, and people say it looks great for my age, especially the wear and tear of the years on camera. I'm telling you, it's my routine. Even if I am dead tired, I will wash my face and apply moisturizer.

I often try new products, and I follow the directions to a T and give them sixty to ninety days as a testing window. For RE/SHAPE, I'm always on the lookout for new hero products—those products none of us should be without. A few years ago, I was introduced to Dr. Nayan Patel, one of the top formulators in the world. He created Auro Skincare, a skincare line that contains the highest form of a kind of antioxidant called *glutathione*. Within twenty-four hours after I tried it the skin on my face actually felt thicker. His revive and reset cream has become a regular part of my weekly routine. After months of pleading with him, we now have it available through our RE/SHAPE shop.

We know our skin changes over the years. It's about creating a routine to serve your needs at that particular time in your life. I always say, start by washing your face. Do you know how many women don't wash their face at night? I love my nighttime face routine; I go to bed oiled up from the top of my forehead all the way down to the top of my chest. Just think about it: you will be sleeping for eight hours, so it's the perfect time for those products to activate and reduce wrinkles, clear blemishes, or reduce puffiness. The products you use are important—the more natural the better. Find your best cleanser, toner, oils, scrubs, masks, and moisturizers. You can use different products on different days. Listen to your skin and feed it what it needs.

Who doesn't love a facial or a special beauty treatment? I am a regular with my aesthetician. I try to go once per month. If once per month is not feasible for you, go every other month, every quarter, twice a year—just go. There are so many great service providers and packages now in this area that this important part of self-care is totally doable. I've been working with Beverly Hills Rejuvenation Center, a nationwide anti-aging and med spa specializing in the most cutting-edge noninvasive beauty treatments. RE/SHAPE has a partnership with BHRC, and I have been working with the owners Dan and Devin to explore and learn about the latest technology to hit the market for the med-spa industry. I love when I receive a call from Dan telling me that they are launching a new service and I'm invited to come test it out. There are so many options now to keep ourselves looking the way we want without going under the knife or shooting too much into our face. Do the research, ask the questions, and learn what is available near you. If you live near a Beverly Hills Rejuvenation Center, give them a call and tell them I sent you!

For my makeup, I love to mix and match. I'm not a one-product-line girl. Finding the right concealer is a must, especially for me because I have dark circles under my eyes. I also love a tinted moisturizer—this is my go-to on days I am not working. It has the perfect coverage; I can add a little mascara and gloss and I'm out the door for carpool, grocery shopping, or whatever is on the to-do list that day.

Over the years, I have found a specific lip pencil, lipstick, and gloss that combined give me my perfect red lip. I've learned how to do my eyes by following the natural bone structure and applying liners and shadows in spots that accentuate my features. The same goes for the other areas of my face. I know the shades and colors that work well on me and how certain product lines serve throughout the day. This part of our beauty routine we need to keep up with as we age. Times change and we change. We need to stay aware of how we are applying our makeup—our eye makeup shouldn't look like it did in our high school senior photo.

There are so many tutorials online to learn about application and choosing colors. This is where it all starts. Get creative, move out of your comfort zone, and try a new color of liner or put on lashes more than just on a special occasion. Build up your makeup routine so it is practical, meets your budget, and, most importantly, makes you feel great about yourself.

What to Wear

I love working with my longtime makeup artist, stylist, and friend Davia. We pair well together because we have always naturally used the *high-low method* for our wardrobe. I love a designer piece as much as the next girl, but I also love finding vintage boots or a cute summer dress at Target. It's how you put it together, and it's the *you* shining through that makes the statement.

Perhaps you need a little update with your wardrobe, or you need some lessons on how to pair your tops and bottoms or how to choose the perfect statement piece for your look. Whatever it is, the support is out there. There are more fashion magazines than we can count; many department stores have stylists working the floor whom you can ask, and I'm sure there is a stylist in your area with whom you can book time so they can identity your body type and make suggestions for how to dress and play up your features.

For me, I have a long torso, so pants that are high-waisted look great. I can also pull off a big pattern from head to toe, whereas someone who doesn't have my height may not carry it off as well. You need to dress for you and what God gave you. Figure out your favorite features and work from there. My best advice to inspire a reshape with your wardrobe is to find another woman whose look you are inspired by and ask for her help to create your own version. I don't know one woman who would say no to that if someone asked her. After all, we are here to be a community for each other so we can live out our best lives.

How good do you feel when you have your look on point? It's a feeling we should have more than once or twice a month, or, gosh, once or twice a year. If you can simplify your wardrobe, know what works for you, fill your closet with the pieces you love and that fit you well, you will be excited to open the doors of your closet every day and create a custom-designed look that is all you!

And remember—our beauty does shine from within. Have you met those people who radiate so much light that you hardly take notice of what they might be wearing or how their hair is done? That is the person I strive to be, where my inner light and how I share it with the world is one of my best features. Don't settle for baggy shirts or the old makeup staples. You are worth every effort to give yourself the gift of a beauty reshape.

RESHAPE WRAP-UP

Vera was skilled at giving the most amazing facials, and her knowledge about the skin was unmatched. Her true gift, though, which I value the most, was compassion and service to others. By treating people with dignity and making them feel seen no matter who they were, she helped so many women discover their true radiance. I believe we can all be inspired to make an impact like that in our own way.

Your routines in self-care and wellness from the inside out are an opportunity to honor yourself in an intimate and purposeful way.

Custom design a beauty reshape with your skincare, with your makeup, with your wardrobe. Make purposeful and informed decisions about how you are enhancing your beautiful features.

RESHAPE MOVES

1. Show yourself the love and compassion you show others. The perfect time for this is when you look in the mirror cleansing your skin, applying your makeup, or checking out your final look before you walk out the door. Resist the urge to be critical of yourself.

2. Find the beauty in other women. Show them compassion and love the way Vera did. Look past their exterior and search their hearts. Be the kind of woman who lifts other women up rather than tearing them down. Even though we

are all different, we can always find something that connects us.

3. Keep your eyes open for the people in your life who feel like sunshine, and keep them close. They will most likely be the same people who see your superpowers.

CHAPTER 9

RESHAPE YOUR BODY

Find What Works for You

Exercise because you love your body,
not because you hate it.

JULIA BUCKLEY

I welcome change in my life because change leads to transformation. I welcome the little bit of stress and slight anxiety that comes with trying new things—it makes me feel alive. New adventures are an opportunity to overcome fear; leave what is familiar, safe, and comfortable; and experience something new. In new situations you have to rise to the occasion and embrace the unknown. You have to surrender.

Though I've been athletic all my life, honestly, running has never been my go-to sport. But when the Boys and Girls Clubs of America asked me to support them by running in the Boston Marathon, I said yes right away. They were inviting me to push into the unknown in search of growth and transformation. Running a marathon had been on my bucket list, and it was for a good cause. I looked forward to the adventure.

I was in pretty good shape at the time, but I wasn't a runner. I'd never run 26.2 miles, so I knew it wasn't going to be easy. The Boston Marathon isn't easy by anyone's standards. So I worked with a trainer to come up with a plan. Then I trained for weeks, logging enough miles to feel confident that I could complete the grueling run. I wasn't super concerned with my time. I just wanted to be able to finish!

With the "Real" Runners

Because I was representing the Boys and Girls Clubs of America, I got to line up at the starting line with the most serious accomplished runners. These were the world-class marathoners, people who'd run multiple marathons—who *lived* to run them. One guy I talked with had flown in from Kenya. He'd run the Boston multiple times and was determined to beat his previous time. When he told me what his record time was, my jaw dropped. I couldn't believe I would be running with this guy. I was completely green, doing it for the adventure and for the Boys and Girls Club.

There are so many runners that the whole thing takes hours to get started. We waited at the starting line, stretching and trying to stay loose. When it was finally go-time, I was so excited I sprinted, but I quickly fell behind. My fellow runners at the start were so fast! I nearly ran into a ditch letting the faster runners pass.

Donut Detour

After I'd been running for about an hour, I felt the strong urge to go to the bathroom. I'd heard stories of people having accidents while running. I was not about to let that be me. The route had taken us into a suburban area. All along the road people gathered, cheering us on with signs and even water for thirsty runners. I hadn't seen any of the portables around and I really had to go, so I asked one of the spectators, "Is there a restroom?" She yelled back, "You can use mine! It's right here!"

So I got out of the pack and followed her into her home close by. When I came out, she had Krispy Kreme donuts sitting on the table. She offered me one, and I couldn't resist; I sat right down and ate my donut at the kitchen table. Then we started chatting. I was telling her about my family and complimenting how cute her kitchen was, just having the best time, when suddenly it hit me. I said, "The race! Oh no! I have to go!"

By the time I got back into the race, most of the runners were long gone. There were only a few of the slowest runners at the very tail end. I'd gone from being in the front with the world-class athletes, to meeting this wonderful woman with her Krispy Kreme donuts, to running at the tail end of the race. There was pretty much nobody else around—no more spectators cheering us on. Just myself and a handful of others.

I kept at it. When I crossed the finish line, I didn't bother to check my time. I knew I hadn't broken any records. I later learned that it took me five hours and forty-one minutes to run those 26.2 miles. For reference, the record for fastest Boston Marathon is two hours and three minutes. Even so, I felt really proud of myself. I'd set a goal for myself to finish, I'd had an incredible experience, and I could check "Boston Marathon" off my bucket list.

It had been a huge challenge. There were many, many times when I wondered, *Can I really do this?* But I stepped outside my comfort zone and pushed the boundaries of what I'd known to be possible. Every time I have done this in my life, I have experienced huge growth—and now I have a great story too.

Finding What Works

Even after having grown up in team sports, running the Boston Marathon taught me things about myself that hold true to this day. I hope these things can help you find what works when figuring out how to move your body and explore a fitness reshape for yourself.

- **People.** I'm such a people-person that I know I'm more likely to participate and enjoy moving if I have the promise of good company. It also helps to have someone cheering me on and holding me accountable.
- **Adventure.** If I schedule time to get on the treadmill and zone out, I'm going to dread it. But when I make a date to do

something new and fun, I get excited and I'm more likely to show up with enthusiasm. When I frame my fitness as "adventure," I find that makes it more fun.

- **Goals.** I'm naturally competitive with myself and love working toward goals. By choosing fitness activities that tap into the way I am naturally wired, I ensure I won't ever get burned out or bored.

I've learned a lot about what works for my body in the years since the marathon. And my body is constantly changing, so I like to explore new ways to move, discovering each day what works best for me. These days I love getting out for a hike, going for walks with friends in my neighborhood, going to cardio classes. The important thing is to make fitness activities something I enjoy.

Sure, I am always hoping the result is me dropping a few pounds or tightening my booty, which seems to be sitting on the back of my thighs these days, but really it's about how I feel afterward. Even if I do a fifteen-minute stretch session, I am moving, checking in with my body. When I move daily it changes my mindset. I feel accomplished; I feel happier. No matter where I am on my fitness journey I know that I am doing what it takes to get me one step closer to my goal, whether it's losing those few extra pounds or building better mobility. A consistent routine is key.

As my friend Robin Sharma points out, the daily benefits of cardio are so incredible that it's amazing more people don't take advantage of them. "Sweating releases BDNF, a brain chemical that actually grows neural connections. Working out also releases dopamine (the neurotransmitter of motivation) and serotonin, which makes you feel happy."[6]

I am always switching up my routines to keep things fresh, but my main goal is to always move with intention every single day.

Prioritizing the Time

I may feel down some days, but as soon as I move my body the endorphins are set free and I am good again.

As women, a huge barrier to fitness is often guilt. When it comes to self-care, it's easy to think that we should be using that time to attend to the kids or a task on our never-ending to-do list. When we're busy, self-care is easily the first thing to go.

But years ago my mom said something I'll never forget. She said, "If we don't take care of ourselves, no one else will." It's true, and I think of that often. I've learned that when I show up for myself, I have so much more energy for my children, my husband, and my work. By caring for me I am able to care for them better.

I am happier, more confident, and nicer to my family when I take time to care for my body. It's not just a gift to myself; it's a gift to those around me. When I release those endorphins, serotonin, and dopamine—all essential happiness chemicals—I'm not just helping myself, I'm sharing the joy! Taking the time to exercise isn't just about the way our clothes fit; it's about feeling great in your body, mind, and spirit.

What does this staying fit look like for me?

Taking care of myself doesn't mean me first, it means me too.

L. R. Knost

Making Space

Most days I love to work out. I feel so good after making the effort to get in cardio, a class, a weight-training session, or even a stretch. Year after year, I find it more necessary to stay consistent with my fitness routine because it is foundational for me to live my best life.

But there are those days, of course, when I would rather just lounge—and sometimes I do.

My schedule before lockdown included taking a couple of classes every week and scheduling workouts with my neighborhood friends, but when the pandemic hit, that shut down with everything else. The question became, how do I maintain my fitness routines?

Every inch of our house was maxed out, especially with kids doing school from home. Even with all the change to our daily flow, I knew it was necessary to set myself up so I could at the very least find thirty minutes to move my body every day.

I put together a simple fitness kit with my basics—three- and five-pound hand weights, ankle weights, a yoga mat, and a resistance band and sliders—that I use to elevate my workouts in the most powerful way. Each fitness tool is purposeful, even my wardrobe choices. Creating a space in the corner of my bedroom where I can keep everything neatly in a basket has made a huge difference with my mindset. I have everything ready, so there's no need to think. Anytime I can give myself the gift of thirty minutes, I can jump right in and I don't give the space to talk myself out of it.

Now that I'm prepped and organized, I'm more likely to stay on track when I feel that urge to lounge rather than sweat. I know that if a class is booked, I can always work out at home, take a hike with the kids, or walk the dog in the neighborhood. I always like to have options available.

Workout Basics

Signing up for a gym can be great, but it's not right for everyone. I've had my fair share of gym memberships, but working out at home is always more convenient. I set up an area in my home that works perfectly well for fitness routines. It's not a whole room, just a clear space in front of my desk. I really only need a little area to do my entire workout.

If you're just getting started, I'd encourage you to wear something you feel good in—maybe a cute new workout outfit. Can you exercise in a T-shirt and a pair of old shorts? Sure! I just know that for me, it inspires me when I have something nice to exercise in. I feel more together. And again, it's a reminder that you're worth it!

Because of my injuries, I am constantly working around pain, and sometimes a workout activates it. I have now figured out what those triggers are, and I know how to make modifications. The important thing is to never stop moving my body and stretching.

Stretching has become a powerful part of pain management for me. I used to think stretching was for "older people." Now I look at it as the saving grace when it comes to caring for my body!

As far as equipment, keep it simple. All I really need is my set of ankle weights, a set of resistance bands, and a three- or five-pound weight. I also love having a mirror nearby so I can watch my form. When I travel, I bring a set of Bala Resistance Bands and Bala Sliders. That way I have everything I need to do an amazing workout, and I don't ever need to go to the gym.

Schedule It and Honor It

With my busy life, I live by a schedule. At different seasons of the year, I have to reshape my schedule, and that is okay. Getting movement in every day looks different no matter where I am or what's going on. At the start of each week, I sit down with my calendar and plan out my week. I know if I don't plan for it, it won't happen. That's why I set aside time to exercise daily. I don't apologize for it. If someone asks for that time slot, I say, "That time isn't available. What other time will work for you?"

I enjoy going to classes and working out in groups, but there are so many great online classes and videos that it's really easy to work out at home. Or just take a walk in the neighborhood or go on a bike ride. The main thing is making sure to move every day. For me, movement, exercise, and confidence go hand in hand. When I exercise I can see my confidence building because I know I am doing something just for me, and that feels really good. Honoring this part of my life has affected all areas of my heart, mind, soul, and health. It's amazing how with thirty minutes a day of movement, at whatever level you might be, can create meaningful improvements across your entire life.

I don't do this perfectly. Some days I fall short. But if I miss a day of exercise, the next day I get back at it. Consistency is key with fitness just as it is in any area of life where you desire results.

———————— RESHAPE WRAP-UP ————————

Fitness is not just about fitting into your favorite pair of jeans, although that is great. Fitness is about taking personal control of our health on a daily basis. It is the one area where we can decide what happens from day to day. And that decision will affect every area of our lives for all our future days.

Every single part of your body in enhanced by movement and exercise. Movement for at least thirty minutes a day leads to a reduction in inflammation, it strengthens and tones all your muscles, and it releases stress and anxiety.

Our bodies and our health are a gift. Keeping up with a good fitness schedule is the ultimate way to honor ourselves.

Fitness is the best way to challenge yourself, your mental toughness, your tenacity as a person, your dedication, and your consistency to accomplish a goal.

RESHAPE MOVES ─────────────

1. Schedule it. Set aside a time. Don't just assume you will fit it in at some point during your day. Schedule your exercise at least a week out so any meetings or daily responsibilities can be scheduled around it.

2. Find fitness systems and activities you love and are energized by. This will keep you motivated to stay with it.

3. Make it convenient. Have your workout clothes washed and ready. Put your shoes on in the morning.

4. Figure out the accountability you need. Do you need to meet up with friends for a walk or a class? Do you need to invest in hiring a trainer? Do you need to track your progress through an app? You know you. Put a system in place that serves your goals, and stick with it. Keep your goal in mind. I often write a goal on a sticky note and place it on the mirror in the bathroom. I've even been known to write it in lipstick.

CHAPTER 10

RESHAPE YOUR MINDSET

What You Think Determines

How You Feel

The way you tell your story to yourself matters.

AMY CUDDY

Becoming a wellness explorer opened my eyes to the possibilities of vibrant health. Like so much in life, vibrant health begins with mindset. Somehow this idea has always been with me, even when I was young and unsure of how to give voice to it. After all, I'd utilized mindset and visualization in the bathtub years ago, and that yielded my life's first true reshape moment at the Miss USA competition.

I've heard it said that the quality of your thoughts is the quality of your life. That statement, in my experience, has been absolutely true! In a very real way, what we think affects every aspect of being.

One of my favorite Bible verses is, "All things are possible to him who believes" (Mark 9:23 NKJV). If you can't tell by now, inspirational quotes and solid strategies have been the building blocks for my life. Are you a person who looks at the glass half full or half empty? Are you a person with a "can do" mindset? However you approach life is the life you will have.

I truly believe establishing a particular mindset for how you are going to approach your life is the foundation for everything. That's true whether everything is sunny days and ocean breezes in your mind or if you are up against a wall dealing with pressure so strong you feel you might break. Your mind is the most powerful tool you have. Your view of yourself and the world around you will dictate your day-to-day and your future.

You are in control. You are in control of what you do, and you are in control of how you engage and respond to anything outside yourself. How we see ourselves, how we internalize our thoughts and feelings, creates the pattern for how we move through life.

Mindset is not the easiest reshape by any means. But the way we handle our internal dialog with ourselves is the driver of our lives. How is your self-talk? Are you speaking life into yourself daily? Do you start that day with an "anything is possible" attitude and believe that you can accomplish your goals and dreams?

We've all traveled different roads, and I recognize there are times in life when just getting up each day is about all you can do. I believe, however, that if you work to condition your mindset during the good times, the more difficult times don't last as long and you'll find your way out.

I can assure you that you can manifest your dreams. You can make real what you see in your mind's eye for your life. You can create a life you love. It all starts with faith, belief in yourself, and an unwavering mindset.

I naturally see the glass half full. But I wanted to educate myself on a deeper level. An opportunity came up for me to attend a leadership and growth conference in Los Angeles, and I was excited to learn. There I heard from authors, coaches, and scientists, which gave me a road map to explore new frontiers of my mindset. That weekend I connected with a group who'd put together a trip to climb Mount Fuji as a manifestation of all that we had been inspired by at the conference.

They asked me to come along.

When they proposed this trip, as wild and impromptu as it was, something in me said yes immediately, with no planning, and I stepped over my fear. Admittedly, I love an adventure. And climbing Mount Fuji in Japan, the thirty-fifth largest mountain in the world at over 12,000 feet, was definitely adventurous. I had never climbed a mountain, but I longed to hike outside my comfort zone and test my limits. I sensed that outside those limits I would experience growth. Would I have thought up this adventure on my own? Probably not. But the opportunity had been handed to me. This group was going to do all the planning. All I had to was commit, dip into my rainy-day savings, and show up. As Constantine Dhonau, author of *Collateral Intentions*, might put it, I was "surrendering to the current of life."[7]

I was all in.

Now, to be clear, this was not a sightseeing trip. The total focus was scaling Mount Fuji. The plan was to fly to Japan, get a good night's sleep, then head to the mountain, climb all day, sleep on the mountain, summit at sunrise, then make our way down and leave the following day. That's a lot of miles to cover in a short time. But again, I was excited and I was up for it.

Laser Focus

As soon as I said yes my mind became laser focused. Preparing was part of getting into the right mindset—thinking through what would be needed. I headed to my local REI and geared up. I got the headlamp, the water bladder to wear, a good backpack, hiking boots, hiking clothes that were breathable and quick drying like thermal layers, rain gear, and some freeze-dried snacks. This was challenging for me because I am the kind of traveler who normally packs everything but the kitchen sink. I like my suitcase to be like Mary Poppins's bag. If something might be needed, I like to have it on hand. This time, I'd have to pack carefully. I even trained by walking daily on my treadmill at the highest incline with my hiking boots and backpack filled with weights.

Finally the day arrived. I made my way to Japan and then to the mountain. Our ascent began at a hiking station on the lower quarter of the mountain. What amazed me at first was seeing so many groups descending the mountain. Older people, some in their seventies, eighties, maybe even nineties, made their way down with their children and grandchildren. The guides informed us that Mount Fuji is one of Japan's three sacred mountains and has a long history as a religious site for the Japanese. Many make a yearly pilgrimage to this special place. So many of these people were dressed like they'd walked out of their backyard and said, "I think I'll just take a stroll up the mountain today." And there I was in my full hiking gear, brand-new hiking boots, backpack, rain gear, and water bladder with the tube. I was tempted to feel like I'd overdone it. But I reminded myself that we were on a very, very large mountain—the highest in Japan. Along the way, we greeted many more groups of people hiking down. Each time, I thought to myself, *I wonder why they're here.* I couldn't even say for sure why I was there, but I knew I was supposed to be there.

At first, my inner dialog was mundane. Did I have the right gear? Had I prepared adequately? And I had some safety concerns too. At times I'd think, *This is dangerous! My mother won't drive on a freeway without a shoulder, and here I am on the edge of a mountain, thousands of feet in the sky. She would lose her mind if she saw the circumstances I put myself in!* My mind was clouded by those thoughts at first. The higher I climbed, the more challenging it became. I was completely outside of my element, far removed from my ordinary world. I began to settle in and just put one foot in front of the other. I began to open up to the lessons the climb was teaching and simply be. I was able to cut through the nagging voice in my head: *Do I have enough water? Did I pack my wet/dry blanket? OMG, I have to pee in that hole in the ground? Will there be a bed at the top to sleep on? Is my sock bunching up and giving me a blister? If my mom saw how close I was to the edge she would kill me.* When all that fell quiet, I began to receive the thoughts, the information, the wisdom delivered to me in those moments. I felt an internal shift on that mountain, a receiving of peace and insights.

Insights on the Mountain

I realized that this adventure was a huge gift, especially since I was doing it on my own with a group of strangers. Sometimes being alone is the best thing you can do for yourself. It's a reminder that you don't need your friends, you don't need a spouse, you don't need a partner. Those things are nice, but they're not necessary. Sometimes it's good to get away by yourself and just be with your thoughts until they're clear. I'm not suggesting such times need to be halfway around the world or even out of your hometown! It can happen on a walk in a park or at a coffee shop. The idea is, just being alone with our thoughts can be clarifying. For me this was a profound example of one of those times. Instinctually I think I'd known I needed this adventure.

Each time we reached a hiking station, we got to rest for a moment. The attendants stamped our hiking sticks: 5,000, 10,000, 12,000 . . . I still have that stick with the Japanese flag tied to it, stamped with how high I climbed. How amazing to go so high!

> The earth has music for those who listen.
>
> *Reginald Vincent Holmes*

Then it began to rain. Even in the wet and cold, with the light fading so that we needed headlamps to see, my adrenaline was pumping. I was so excited and proud to be on this adventure. At one of the stations we stopped to eat. Low wooden tables invited us to sit and enjoy a warm meal. I'd only eaten my little freeze-dried snacks, and my body was depleted. I was ravenous! We were served a meal of rice and curry. I ate every bite, and gosh, how I wanted seconds, but they were only giving one plate per person to make sure they had enough for everyone. Even though I could have eaten more, it hit the spot and was warm, nourishing, and comforting—exactly what I needed.

That night we slept on the mountain. We were really high up, and I was soaking wet at that point. We stopped at a shelter where pallets were stacked like bunkbeds. I shed my first layer of wet clothing and pulled something dry out of my pack, tucking myself in tight to get warm. There were no pillows, just a thin mat to lie on. Though there was no heat and I was wet and cold, at least we were sheltered from the wind and rain. I was so exhausted that I fell asleep quickly.

Above the Clouds

We woke while it was still dark and hiked to the mountaintop as the sun rose. As we reached the peak, I realized we were literally above the clouds. I could reach out and run my hands through the mist. I've never seen anything like it. Then the sun came up. I was exhausted, but I tried to let it soak in: I'd done it. I'd climbed Mount Fuji.

Going back down was a whole other adventure. A group of us walked ahead of the rest, but we took a wrong turn. We did not know where we were. Still, it was clear that we were going down so we knew at some point we would arrive at either the bottom of the mountain or some sort of checkpoint station. The strange thing was, we assumed that it would be like it was as we went up—that we'd cross paths with people headed up as we went down. But it was just us—not another soul in sight. We did not run into one single person going down the mountain. Plus, it was a totally different terrain. As we went up it was rocky, with not that much vegetation. Going down it was like we were going through forests and tall grass, and there was a tiny path. I worried, thinking, *Where is everybody?* Once I settled into the idea that obviously we went down the wrong way and we would just have to figure it out at the bottom, I was able to enjoy the journey.

Finally, at the bottom of the mountain there was a new imperative: find a bus station. We were all dirty and stinky and wet, having been hiking for two days. Japan is so pristine and clean, and here came our crew of dirty, stinky American hikers. I'm sure we were quite a sight.

I could barely walk the next day. I was so sore. It was incredibly taxing, around eighteen hours of exertion. Climbing up worked the back of my legs; walking down I worked the whole front part of my legs, so both sides had been put to the test. Even though I could barely walk, I felt incredible. It was awesome, and looking back I'm so happy I did it. Such a great life experience. I crave more experiences like that in my life.

I surrendered myself to what life was handing me—the opportunity that was presented. I could easily have let fear keep me from doing it, but I stepped through it and discovered something profound about myself. My love and passion for adventure, the unknown, and living life to the fullest bloomed in me on that trip. It felt like such a time of growth for me. Being in untamed nature produced energy in me like I had never experienced. I felt so connected, truly submersed in the elements.

I'm so glad I went for it.

My Climb to Pain-Free Living

The car accident I was in more than twenty years earlier challenged me in a totally different way. It wasn't a terribly serious accident; I wasn't hospitalized. But the collision jerked my body around so much that I was never the same.

I continued to live an active, full life after that, but I lived with a consistent, simmering pain in my neck, back, and shoulders. At times, as I've mentioned, I couldn't sleep. Other times I'd experience a piercing pain in my shoulder. My pain tolerance level is pretty high, and with my strong work ethic, I could almost always power through. But when the quality of my life began to be disrupted by pain and I felt powerless against it, I realized I needed help.

I sought out experts. Physical therapists, acupuncturist massage therapists, herbalists, chiropractors, you name it. I experimented with many different modalities, and each time I got some relief from treatment. But that relief was temporary. Instead of progressing into good health, I was getting only temporary pauses on the pain.

Over the years, with each new appointment, I'd feel hopeful. Each time I found a new resource, I'd think, *This is going to be it! We are going to identify my issue, resolve it, and I'll be pain free!* I threw myself at the treatment, giving it my all—my will, resources, energy, and time. I spent countless hours arranging meetings, filling out paperwork, driving to appointments an hour away, and doing all the waiting. Sometimes practitioners required multiple visits in a week. It was a lot, and chasing this pain was consuming my life.

In all honesty, sometimes I felt guilty, wondering if I was wasting time. And much of that time did seem fruitless. I wondered if it was worth the effort. After all, it seemed my pain wasn't signaling a terminal issue. It wasn't going to kill me. I wasn't confined to my home or unable to walk. Many women suffer far worse. Perhaps that was why I didn't complain. I kept my struggle quiet for the most part, but deep inside I knew this was a battle I needed to fight and win.

Self-advocacy has always been an important value for me, instilled in me by my mom. That said, my experience taught me how difficult it can be to speak up for yourself when it comes to your health. It can be incredibly hard! I believe it's why so many of us end up relinquishing our power to healthcare providers instead of fighting for what we deserve. Pursuing options that work for your unique situation takes a lot of willpower. And if you're already feeling compromised and weak, it's doubly trying.

For me, each time I found a new modality or healthcare provider who promised relief, I would be hopeful. Then after five or six sessions, it would hit me: *This is not working.* Sometimes I would cry in frustration and temporary defeat. Did I have the energy to try something else? Would I ever figure this out? But after I pushed through my disappointment, I always knew the answer. *Yes.* It's that mindset of never settling and trying your best to reach your goal, even if you have to figure it out by yourself.

The record player in your mind should be telling you: *I want more for my life, and I don't have to live like this.* The energy we invest in figuring out the areas of life that cause the most challenges will ultimately release the weight in other areas of life that are compensating. Every minute you invest in yourself will come back to you tenfold. Taking that approach to life and becoming the master of your own mindset will lead you through anything.

I struggled for many years until I reached the breaking point that became a turning point. My burnout while filming *Hollywood Today* was a reshape bridge—a blessing I hadn't known to ask for. My crisis had become a quest. That's when I became a wellness explorer and launched RE/SHAPE. I discovered solutions that really work for me. I honestly feel better today than I did twenty years ago. The pursuit of the right combination took decades, but I found it. Has it been a struggle? Yes. Has it been worth it? One hundred percent. Did I have to be patient? Yes! Do I still have flare-ups? Yes, but the amount of time I am not in pain is more than the amount of time I am in pain, so I call that a huge success. I am proud to say that I did not give up on me.

God puts us exactly where we need to be. If I had not experienced that pain for years, I would have not have taken my first steps as a wellness explorer and I would not have started RE/SHAPE. I would not have begun writing this book, sharing my story with you with the hope that my experiences can help you on your own reshape journey.

There is no one-size-fits-all solution when it comes to health or life. Please don't let anyone convince you otherwise. The world tends to put everyone in a box because that works for the system—and for marketing! The truth is that we are each uniquely and wonderfully made. Each of us is a masterpiece in the making.

In a very real way, mindset literally determines the future. If I had given in to nagging thoughts and worries, I'd have robbed myself of the peace, the wisdom, the insights, and the experience of Mount Fuji. If I'd given negativity space in my mind, I'd have given in to doctors who said I'd have to medicate my pain, limit my activities, and just "live with it" unless I wanted to have surgery.

Having a healthy mindset often requires that we say no to negative thoughts. I've taught myself to actively flip the switch on negative thoughts and unhealthy self-talk. Imagine there's a button or dial on those negative thoughts that say you are not good enough, deserving enough, or worthy enough—and just click it to the off position! Negative thoughts will keep you from living your best life. Send them packing.

I don't just eliminate unhealthy thoughts; I actively increase positive thoughts through my day, getting inspiration from quotes, reading great books, surrounding myself with positive people, visualization, and meditation. I also make sure the conversations I engage in come from a place of positivity and good energy. I say no to negativity and gossip. That helps me keep my mindset healthy, clear, and positive.

Other ways I actively engage a healthy mindset include some things we've discussed already but that work every time to ease my mind:

- **Exercise.** Moving my body always gets me out of a bad mood.
- **Self-care.** Even just the simple act of putting lotion on my body in an act of caring for myself pulls me a little farther out of the funk.
- **Stepping into the natural world.** Going for a walk in nature, rain or shine, can work wonders for my mindset. I especially love digging my hands in the soil, weeding or pruning plants in the garden or foraging in the yard or neighborhood for arrangements for the house. Putting something good and healthy in my body often changes my mindset too.

Setting exciting goals and believing you are capable of achieving them is part of living the life of your dreams. This does take consistent daily practice. We don't change anything overnight, especially an embedded way of thinking about ourselves or the world.

Giving Yourself Space to Pivot

Several years ago, my friend Gail Becker, creator of Caulipower, was at the very top of her industry in public relations and marketing. She worked on some of the most notable corporate ad campaigns that we have all seen over the years, and she was on the communications teams of some successful politicians. She'd worked hard and was reaping the benefits of her efforts. She had all the trappings of success, but she wasn't feeling satisfied. Something in her knew there was more to life.

Gail decided to exit her job and launch her own business. She went from a successful executive in PR and marketing to starting a plant-based pizza company. Today Gail's company is one of the hottest in the country. She's won numerous awards and accolades and now is thriving not only in her business but deep down in her soul. Gail will be the first one to tell you that she was scared, didn't know how she was going to do it, and faced a steep learning curve, but she knew who she was and what she was capable of, so she doubled down, kept her eye on the prize, and made it happen.

Maybe It's Time for You to Change Your Mind

Your mindset reshape doesn't have to be a huge career shift like Gail's. It could possibly show up as learning a new skill or getting certified in something you feel gifted at. Maybe it's serving in the community or just being there for a friend or acquaintance who needs your encouragement and help.

Are you fulfilled? What needs to change? Are you willing to take the risk to receive the reward? If you are truly not happy deep within, you can make that choice to take steps to reshape the area of your life that is no longer serving you. You can be happy; you can be fulfilled; you can create a life you love. Mindset is the key—it all starts there. Your mindset can either stop you or propel you; it's your choice.

If you begin to take the necessary steps, even just one at a time, to achieve your goals, change your worldview, or change how you feel about yourself, the complete empowerment you will feel will be a total reset for your life. It's amazing that when you choose to make one small improvement in any area of your life, the state of your mind, heart, and soul begins to change and reshape almost immediately. It's the best feeling! Money can't buy it, no one can give it to you as a gift, you cannot borrow it—it's all you and your determined spirit not to settle and to build the best version of you.

Meet the Expert: Dr. Henry Cloud

Change is an inevitable part of life. There are changes we plan for and others we don't. Any *intentional* reshape necessitates positive change. That's why I loved spending time with the world-famous Dr. Henry Cloud. He has a great way of talking about change. This is a mindset that will serve us all well. He breaks change down into a doable process. If you're in the midst of change right now or are planning a reshape of your own, check out these five steps.

Five Steps to Positive Change

1. **Vision.** To change, you need to get clear about what you want. There's gotta be a *why* and a vision. "I'm here, and I want to be there." Once you're clear about that, you've begun.

2. **Team.** You're probably not going to get where you want to be by yourself. You need to put your team together. Who you choose to be on your team is up to you. It could be a friend, it might be a mentor, it might be a trainer or a coach—but this person or these people

should give you the fuel, energy, and intelligence that can help you along this path.

3. **Plan.** A plan is a strategy for how to make it happen. The plan includes steps—actions or activities—that you actually execute. You can't just go out and suddenly find yourself at your goal. You need a plan. And, by the way, don't just make it up. Find a proven plan—one that has gotten results before.

4. **Measure.** It's important to hold yourself accountable to your vision. Once you're working the plan, be accountable to your team, whoever that is. You need someone who will care if you're getting where you said you wanted to go. Measure to see if you are making progress, and if not, ask why. Work on the obstacles. Tweak the plan as needed.

5. **Adapt.** As soon as you start to measure and get the answer, you have to quickly adapt and fix that.[8]

That's it! Start with a vision, get your team together, create a plan with steps, measure and hold yourself accountable, adapt as needed.

Daydreaming

Growing up in Louisiana, my siblings and I were given free rein to play outside and use our imaginations. With the soybean truck as our swimming pool, the trees as our castles, and the trampoline as our circus tent, we daydreamed our days away, playing in the old barn or our "archaeological dig" site.

I dreamed about where I could go outside my little town. I dreamed of having a family. I dreamed of traveling the world and having the most incredible life experiences.

Don't be scared to dream. You may hesitate because you feel your dreams could never come true and you don't want to set yourself up for disappointment. But what if they do come true? What if you can live out your dream in some way? You are never too old to dream and visualize yourself living the life you want. If you don't daydream and spend time thinking about your future, how do you know where you are going?

When we daydream, we say no to stress and anxiety and say yes to peace and creativity. Those daydreams often become our reality. This really is about living with intention and purpose. Daydreaming can take you away from the day-to-day hustle of life, but it is an important underlying element for how you reach your full potential. What we think about, we create for our lives. Our mindset can change our situations. The mental pictures we create for our lives are the customized blueprints to building growth and living an inspired life—the life we have literally dreamed of.

> The biggest adventure you can ever take is to live the life of your dreams.
>
> *Oprah Winfrey*

Sometimes if I'm feeling stressed or overwhelmed, I imagine the white hallways of my mind and I use my mental "blower" to clear them out. I perceive the light from the sun coming in and flowers starting to grow, and I feel lighter, clearer.

The daydream sequence of resetting your mindset works to

release stress when you feel overwhelmed. Daydreaming is the gateway to reshaping your mindset for the areas of your life you want to focus on. I read a book by Ken Abraham, an influential businessman in the addiction recovery space. He titled his book *Believable Hope*. The title of that book is deep when you think about it. If you have believable hope in your mind and you let your dreams lift you to where you want to go, there is nothing you cannot see or do or experience. A changed mind can lead you on an extraordinary adventure called *your life*!

Mindset Inspirations

Here are some ideas that have worked to help me keep a positive mindset; I hope they work for you.

Vision Board It

Set up a Pinterest "dream board" to inspire yourself! As I've said, I enjoy Pinterest, so I use that app as a vision board. I do this for every area of my life. I shared with you that in building our little beach house in Mexico, I had been creating a vision board of what this home would look like for years before it was even possible to do it on Pinterest. When the time came, I was well on my way to creating my dream space. I have conditioned my mind to live in expectation with all things. So when the opportunity came for us to build our place, it was further evidence of both the practical and having faith. Gratitude naturally followed; as the verse says, when we take delight in God, he gives us the desires of our hearts (Psalm 37:4). But it all starts with our mindset, and it depends on whether we can see it and truly believe it for ourselves.

Say Thanks

The first thing I do when I open my eyes each day is say *thank you*. I name at least three things I'm grateful for, and then I say a simple prayer to affirm how I want to show up in the world.

Keep a Gratitude Diary

I journal daily, and I often list things I'm grateful for. Sometimes I list simple things like my health, or that I can walk, that I have a roof over my head, that I am able to provide food for my family. Other times I express gratitude for an experience I had or a person who entered my life unexpectedly. You will find that as you start to think about all of the things in your life you can be grateful for, the list goes on and on, almost to eternity. With gratitude present in your life, negativity and depression dissipate. And as Steve Harvey says, "if you are grateful for what you have, you open the pipeline for more to come in."[9] I've seen it. In fact, now I am almost fearful that if I lack gratitude, it will block blessings from coming in. Gratitude is the armor I walk into my day with. It protects me from negativity.

Share the Love

Speak out compliments, encouragement, and love to others. Don't hold it back! When you withhold a kind thought or smile or compliment, you are holding back a precious gift that has the potential to change someone's life. Speak it freely! Sincerely give them that gift. I've never forgotten the time a childhood friend was visiting me in Los Angeles and, after spending the day with me and my three-year-old, he said, "You are a really good mom." Something so simple meant the world to me. I teach this to my kids. A kind thought was delivered to you for a reason, so it is your responsibility to give it away.

Sharing your love with others can do wonders for loving yourself and improving your mindset. We see ourselves in others. You can uniquely feel others based on your experience. Often what we need the most in our lives, we need to give to others. Love is reciprocal—either within ourselves or through others.

Meditate

Research continues to show that meditation is excellent for our health. It doesn't really matter exactly how you do it. I try to find at least five minutes in the morning to sit in a quiet place to light a candle—or preferably for fifteen minutes or more when I can. It's an opportunity to experience a different way of perceiving myself and my life before my day gets filled up. I sit in silence or listen to a peaceful playlist, breathing deliberately. I start with a prayer. I practice clearing my mind of clutter, emptying out all my worries, fears, insecurities, to-do lists. Sometimes I move my body as needed, stretching, praying to God for what my heart and soul desires in as much detail as possible, asking him to fill me back up with what I need to move forward into my day. Sure, I get distracted by thoughts coming in, but then I put my focus back on the breath.

You'll be amazed at what happens when you consciously empty out yourself to let God in to work in your life. For me, it helps to read something contemplative, something that feeds my soul, and then I end by journaling on what I've been reading, making note of what was delivered to me in my prayer and meditation.

Initially I was intimidated by meditation. I am so type-A that I didn't even want to try until I knew exactly how to do it. I even went so far as to interview Light Watkins, author of *Bliss More*, so I could learn everything I could before I even tried. We talked about meditation as an eyes-closed, seated practice of focusing. But for some it can be prayer or knitting or some other activity that brings you fully into the present moment with no thought of the past or the future. When we can do that—simply being instead of doing—there is a wonderful carryover into the rest of the day. In fact, you can access that presence and peace when you need it the most, during challenges or struggles.

I started with one of the many apps that offer guided meditation, then my husband joined in, creating a beautiful playlist of Gregorian chants and music that allowed our minds to quiet. Again, it is different for everyone. Our children respect this quiet time, or they join in, sitting in silence beside us.

The definition of mindset is the established attitudes held by someone, a set of beliefs that shape how you make sense of the world and yourself. Mindset influences how you think, feel, and behave, in any given situation.

Do you have an abundance mindset where you find ways to create opportunities and solutions? Do you have a positive mindset, defined as spending more time finding the solution than ruminating on the problem? Do you have a growth mindset, which is a learning mindset and the belief that you can improve—that it's never too late to reshape your life?

Get real with yourself. You know how you think, you know where you have an attitude, and you know how certain mindsets can creep in and cause chaos with your emotions. You know how you feel when you are at your best. Your mindset is yours; make your life soar to the highest levels possible. You have everything within you to do it.

———————— RESHAPE WRAP-UP ————————

We either make ourselves miserable, or we make ourselves strong. The amount of work is the same. Discipline, consistency, and perseverance will take you places motivation never could.

Identify daily habits that will support your forward-thinking, uncluttered mindset. My favorites are exercise, encouraging others, creating a morning and night routine, and not getting wrapped up in drama that has nothing to do with me.

True mental self-care is not a spa day or a once-a-year vacation. It's making choices each day to create a life you don't need to regularly escape from.

Surrender isn't a one-time event. It is a daily choice. Set yourself up with the tools and support you need to consistently make that daily choice.

RESHAPE MOVES ————————————————

1. For two weeks, take notes and observe what story your mind is telling you at the beginning and end of each day. What are you telling yourself throughout the day? Was your mindset full of joy and gratitude? Did you observe your day as exhausting? Mundane? Exciting? Review these thoughts and use them as a baseline to become aware of your mindset. Awareness is always the first step for change.
2. Become self-disciplined about:
   • Meeting your own deadlines
   • Doing the final rep at the gym
   • Making healthy dinners every night

- Turning off your phone or TV at a set time
- Reading a self-help book even when you don't feel like it

3. According to Dr. Caroline Leaf, "if you struggle with overthinking, toxic rumination, self-blame, and intrusive thoughts, you are not alone." Everyone struggles with these things to some degree. Don't feel guilty or ashamed. Your thoughts are valid but not always true. There is hope for overcoming all this. In her latest clinical trials she found that "it takes sixty-three days to unwire toxic thinking habits and trauma from the brain."[10] So stick with it!

CARTWHEELS ON A BEACH

Don't wait for everything to be perfect
before you start enjoying your life.

JOYCE MEYER

For years I'd been dreaming up a trip with my girlfriends where we'd go to an exotic location and experience adventure, pampering, and lots of laughs. So, for my big fortieth birthday, a handful of my oldest friends and I cleared our schedules for a trip to celebrate. As we began making plans, all of a sudden, surprise! I found out I was pregnant! I calculated the due date. It turned out I was basically going to give birth to our third child on my birthday. My birthday gift that year was my baby boy, Valentin, born on the eleventh, ten days before my fortieth birthday—the best birthday gift I have ever received.

I was not about to let this milestone year pass without a celebration, so I simply postponed for a year. That gave me plenty of motivation to stay healthy during my son's first year. Then, on my forty-first birthday, eight girlfriends and I made our way to the Mayan Riviera and Tulum. This was a trip of a lifetime for most of us. We all have so many responsibilities, between families and children and work. I was determined to make the most of it and create an experience we would all remember.

We stayed at the beautiful Grand Velas Resort, right on the beach, owned by a family friend. The girls and I were so excited because we heard that they had the most incredible spa—rated third in the world by *Condé Nast*. We were all thrilled for a little pampering. This weekend was going to be a huge treat.

By now you know how much I love an adventure. I hoped to get us outside of our comfort zones and do new things. I didn't want us to come home with just memories of days spent by the hotel pool, having cocktails, and eating dinner. Those things are fine and good, but my mindset was about celebrating life at forty and our long-lasting friendships.

This was not a passive trip. We stayed active. We did cartwheels in the sand and tried going down into our splits. We stacked up all on top of each other to make pyramids on the beach like we'd done as teenagers. I hadn't felt that way or done some of those things in years, probably since high school. There was a lot of laughter and giggles. We challenged each other to do handstands and float on our backs in the pool for as long as we could, just being silly and having fun.

The region in Mexico where we were staying is known for its spectacular *cenotes*—large sinkholes or caves halfway underground filled with vibrant turquoise water, many of which are connected to a full underground river system. *Cenotes* were considered sacred places by the Mayans, and the fact that we can enjoy this extraordinary manifestation of nature's power, still in the most organic way possible, is amazing to me. It's something I definitely wanted my friends to experience. We zip-lined through and dove down into the cool, deep-blue water. Above us bats hung upside-down among the abundant stalactites. Yes, you read that right: bats. My friends had reservations about that part, but it was all about getting outside our comfort zones, and everyone was game. It was beautiful!

After enjoying the cool water of the *cenotes*, we zip-lined through the trees, which some of us were again nervous about. I don't know if they all enjoyed it in the moment, but I loved every minute of it. We were making memories we'd laugh about for years to come. It gave me joy to know that I was pushing my girlfriends and myself to get outside of the "ordinary" for a while.

We were also guided by a local shaman through a traditional Mayan ceremony. He led us into a cave one by one. It was illuminated by what seemed like hundreds of candles. He burned sage and blessed each of us.

For me, that trip was incredible, filled with the kind of moments that I live for. Stepping out of the day-to-day into a time set aside for new experiences, bonding with friends, expanding my exposure, and reshapes of all kinds, all while beginning a new decade of my life.

Making the Most of the Moment

I am a firm believer in marking occasions and celebrating moments. They mean something in our life. Whether someone plans something for us or we plan something for ourselves, it is important. My encouragement to you is to not let life's moments pass because you feel you don't have time, you don't think you deserve it, or no one is there to mark the occasion with you. The older we get, the more marking these moments matters. They are the building blocks to our lives.

We all come to a point—often it is around middle age—when we begin to look back at the same time we are looking forward. We ask ourselves, how did we get to where we are, and where are we going? The experiences, the life lessons, the decisions, the career paths, our personal lives—all add up to how we establish ourselves in this world.

My memory of this trip and that time in my life provided me with a full opportunity to tap into all the areas we've been talking about in this book: heart, mind, soul, and health. Cartwheels on the beach may not be my everyday life, but it's a snapshot of how I want to walk through life as a whole. We all have so much to be grateful for. If you stop and think, you won't have to go far to realize how much you've got going for you.

Take a look at what you are doing. It is not just about how well you are doing. Ask yourself, *Is this really the best I can do?* The reality is, we don't know about the best we can do, it's so far beyond where we are living.

If you are working to get everything just right before you take that first step to reshape any part of your life, know this: It will probably never be just right. It's the same idea as when you say to yourself, "I will be happy when," fill in the blank: when you get the job promotion, when you lose ten pounds, when you get that new car. Don't wait. It's the right time if you want it to be. You've just got to really want it. You have to have the vision. When you decide you want something, you cannot let your present situation cloud your vision. You might not think you have the resources right in front you; you might think, *I don't have the energy, I don't have the time.* But if you have vision—if you get that picture on the screen of your mind and repeatedly impress it on your heart and in the fiber of who you are—it's going to cause you to act differently and to do the things you need to do to achieve your vision, to attract what you need to help you achieve that goal. Once you make your vision part of you, it's very difficult to let it go and stop making the effort to accomplish it.

You have infinite potential. You have to start with that premise in your mind. You have to really, honestly believe that whatever you want to do, you absolutely can do it if you are willing to do the work. It's not who you are that holds you back; it's who you think you are not. We come up with all kinds of ideas for why we can't do what we really want to do. Quit letting conditions and circumstances control you. It's so easy to get pulled down by what's going on around you. Make up your mind that you are going to flip the switch every time you go there, and move on to thinking about how your dreams can be done.

That comfort zone is a dangerous place to be; it may feel safe, but it's not a good spot to stay in. If your mind can go somewhere, you can physically go there. Everything you want is right here; just grab on to it. You must go out into the unknown. When you go through any fear you face and step toward your dreams, you will have the most amazing experiences in your life. What your heart tells you is far more powerful than what your intellect tells you. Your heart knows the path you should be on. Change your perception; open up to the possibilities. You must create a space in your heart and in your mind for the reshape that you desire. It's the mindset of curating your life.

Nothing stands still; you can never stay where you are. Life is always moving. Are you just putting in time on earth, or are you living? We all have the space to level up our lives, to go deeper and reshape our lives to really live in full color. It all starts with vision, followed by action. Do you really want to sit on the sidelines of your life, or do you want to get in the game and play?

I'm here for you. I'm here cheering you on in this journey. Remember, it's never too late to create a life you love. Don't stand in your own way, and don't settle—because you are worth it all. You are beautiful; let the world see it!

ACKNOWLEDGMENTS

In pure gratitude:

- To my business partner, Rebekah: Thank you for believing in me. I would not have written this book if it wasn't for you. I was fearful to do this project, but you reminded me that on the other side of fear is everything we have ever wanted. Thank you.
- To my cowriter, Amy McConnell; the Fedd Agency; the amazing team at Thomas Nelson; the Lede Company: thank you for holding my hand through this process as a first-time author and for your invaluable contributions at various points in the manuscript.
- To my mother: you have been the greatest example of strength and have instilled in me the belief that anything in life is possible with a dream and hard work.
- To all my friends who I have confided in, laughed and cried with, and who have given me the space to show up with no mask, just as myself: I love you.
- To God's greatest gifts in my life: my husband, Alejandro, and my children, Estela, Marcelo, and Valentin. You are my heartbeat. You inspire me daily to be the best version of myself, and

when I fail you give me grace. I thank you for being my most treasured teachers.

I thank God for walking with me on the journey of this book and giving me the faith to know that it will be exactly what it needs to be for all those who read it. I thank him for helping me to surrender to this process. I ask his forgiveness for the times that I tried to figure out life on my own. I need him to give me direction and wisdom, as I know that his plan is way greater than any plan I can make for myself.

NOTES

1. Oprah Winfrey, "The Powerful Lesson Maya Angelou Taught Oprah," *Oprah's Life Class*, originally aired October 19, 2011, https://www .oprah.com/oprahs-lifeclass/the-powerful-lesson-maya-angelou -taught-oprah-video.
2. Martin Luther King Jr., as quoted by The Martin Luther King, Jr. Center, Twitter post, October 25, 2020, 8:40 a.m., https://twitter.com /thekingcenter/status/1320389731532800000?lang=en.
3. Howard Marks, *The Most Important Thing: Uncommon Sense for the Thoughtful Investor* (Columbia Business School Publishing, 2011), 50–51.
4. John Green, *The Fault in Our Stars* (New York: Penguin, 2014), 286.
5. Joan Moran, "Pause, Reflect and Give Thanks: The Power of Gratitude During the Holidays," *UCLA Newsroom*, October 29, 2013, https://newsroom.ucla.edu/stories/gratitude-249167.
6. Robin Sharma, "The Methods for Superhuman Productivity," *Robin Sharma*, accessed November 28, 2022, https://www.robinsharma .com/article/the-methods-for-superhuman-productivity.
7. Kerry Parsons, interview with Constantine Dhonau, *Chat About Books*, July 26, 2021, https://chataboutbooks.blog/2021/07/26 /authorinterview-with-constantine-dhonau/.
8. Henry Cloud, *Changes that Heal: Four Practical Steps to a Happier, Healthier You* (Grand Rapids: Zondervan, 2009).

9. Steve Harvey, "The Power of Gratitude," YouTube, August 21, 2022, 4:08–4:12, https://www.youtube.com/watch?v=xxXD8fcahMM.

10. Caroline Leaf, "Anyone Else Relate Too Much to This," Facebook, October 17, 2020, https://www.facebook.com/drleaf/photos/anyone -else-relate-too-much-to-this-if-you-struggle-with-overthinking -toxic-rumi/10157374683721078/.

ABOUT THE AUTHOR

After winning Miss USA in 1996, Ali Landry was featured in the iconic Doritos Super Bowl commercial that catapulted her into a successful career as an actress, television host, and brand ambassador. Ali is most proud of her seventeen-year marriage and three beautiful children.

Through her lifestyle brand RE/SHAPE, Ali is committed to researching and curating the best resources, products, and wellness experts to build a community of women who are choosing not to settle and want to level up their lives.

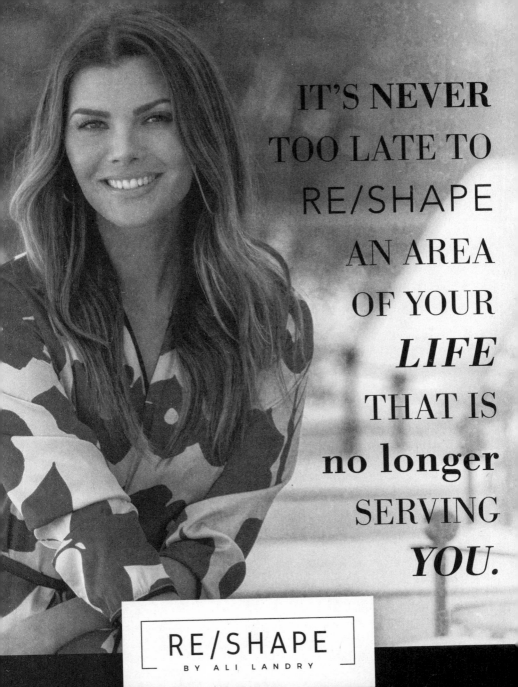